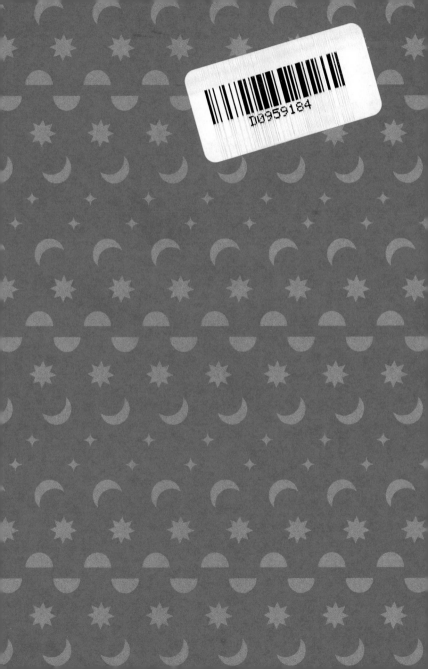

Luminous Dreams

KATIE HUANG

illustrations by BÁRBARA MALAGOLI

Luminous Dreams

EXPLORE THE ABUNDANT
MAGIC AND HIDDEN MEANINGS
IN YOUR DREAMS

CHRONICLE BOOKS
SAN FRANCISCO

Library of Congress Cataloging-in-Publication Data

Names: Huang, Katie, author. | Malagoli, Bárbara, illustrator.
Title: Luminous dreams : explore the abundant magic and hidden meanings
in your dreams / Katie Huang, Bárbara Malagoli.
Description: San Francisco, CA : Chronicle Books, [2022] | Summary: "A
guide to exploring and decoding your dreams"-- Provided by publisher.
Identifiers: LCCN 2022003089 | ISBN 9781797216683 (hardcover)
Subjects: LCSH: Dreams. | Dream interpretation.
Classification: LCC BF1078 .H83 2022 | DDC 154.6/3--dc23/eng/20220308
LC record available at https://lccn.loc.gov/2022003089

Manufactured in China.

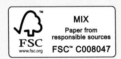

Illustrations by Bárbara Malagoli.
Design by Taylor Roy.

10 9 8 7 6 5 4 3 2 1

Chronicle books and gifts are available at special quantity discounts to
corporations, professional associations, literacy programs, and other
organizations. For details and discount information, please contact our
premiums department at corporatesales@chroniclebooks.com or at
1-800-759-0190.

Chronicle Books LLC
680 Second Street
San Francisco, California 94107
www.chroniclebooks.com

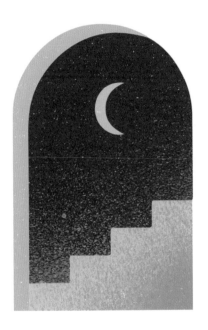

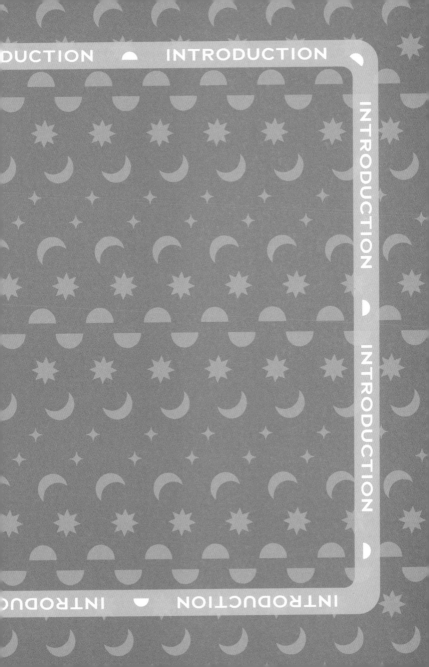

WELCOME, DREAMER.

If you're reading this, you've taken the first step in exploring the mysteries of the dream realm—a place where the subconscious mind is free to wander, the imagination knows no bounds, and infinite possibilities are allowed to bloom. Anything can happen within dreams, which means their potential for healing, growth, and transformation is just as limitless.

Ever since I was a child, I've been fascinated with mystery and the invisible forces of connection that shape our daily lives. Over the past ten years, I've studied and immersed myself in mystical practices and spiritual teachings, and in my experience, some of the most important things in life cannot be measured or explained. Reality isn't just what we can see and touch, but what we feel and know to be true in our hearts. It goes beyond the physical, like intuition and dreams. After all, dreams transcend. They inspire. And like stars, they shine brightest in the dark, illuminating the surrounding shadows and unraveling their secrets.

If you've ever struggled to understand your dreams, or have no idea where to begin, know that I've felt the exact same way. Before I learned how to intuitively interpret my dreams, I had always seen dream interpretation as an elusive practice—one that would usually end in frustration. I'd often look up dream symbols and their meanings online or scour dream dictionaries for information, never once considering that the answers might be within. However, after repeating this process time and time again, I came to realize that by relying upon these external sources rather than my own feelings and perceptions, I had unknowingly disconnected from my greatest source of guidance: my intuition.

I believe that when we harness our intuition, dreams can guide us toward our destiny, acting as a compass for our soul's truth. Sometimes it's easy to trust our intuition. Other times we need a bit of faith. The teachings in this book are designed to help you lean into your inner knowing so that you can embrace your dreams with greater clarity, understanding, and intention. From exploring the reasons why we dream to strengthening your intuitive voice, *Luminous Dreams* will guide you through each step of the dream interpretation process as you connect to deeper states of awareness. I recommend working through this book in chronological order, learning about the basic nature of dreams and intuition first, before moving on to the Intuitive Dream Tool Kit and Intuitive Dream Guide, which discuss practical tools and gentle techniques for dream recall, self-reflection, and better sleep.

As you begin to navigate your dreams, remember: Dream interpretation is not a clear-cut science, but when you follow your intuition you can always find your way home—the way back to yourself.

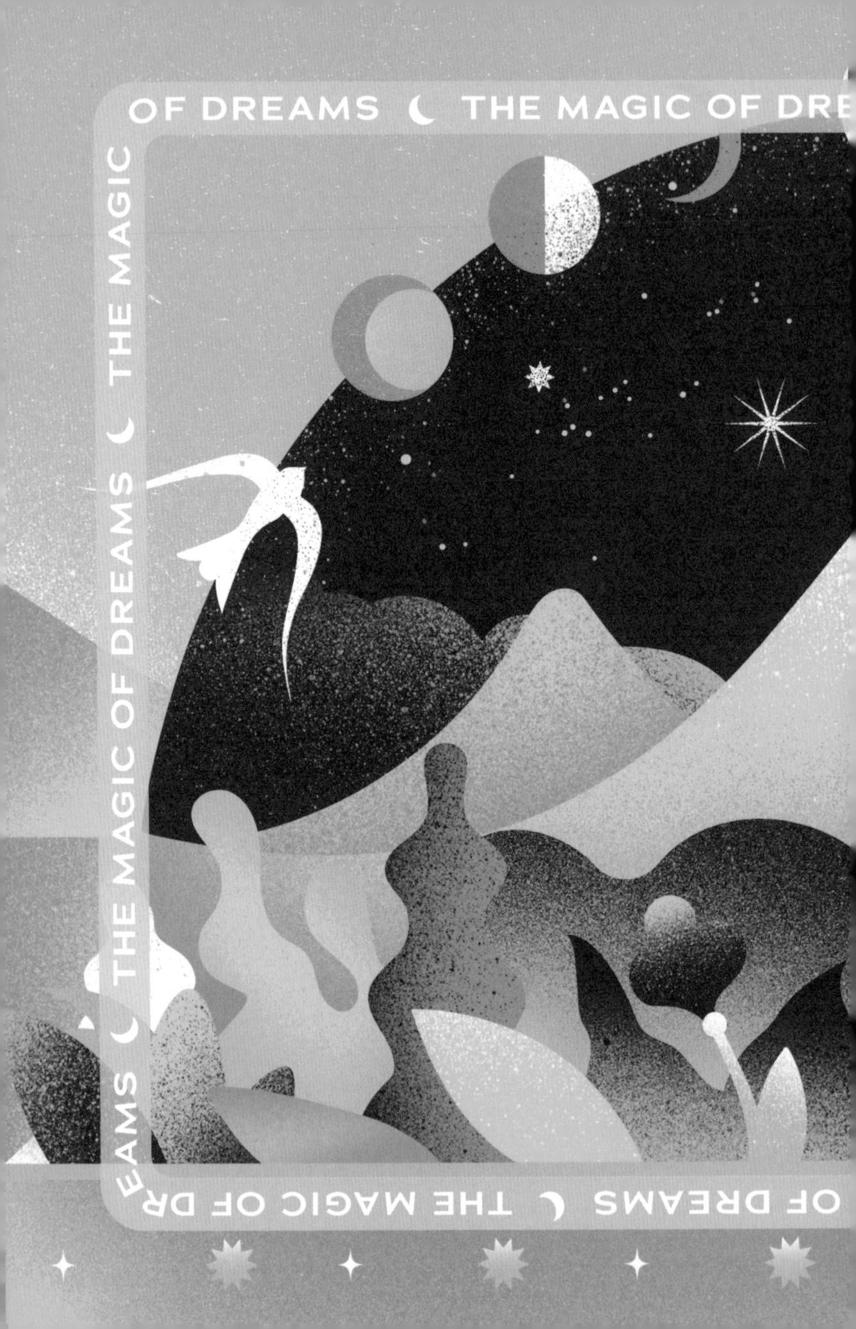

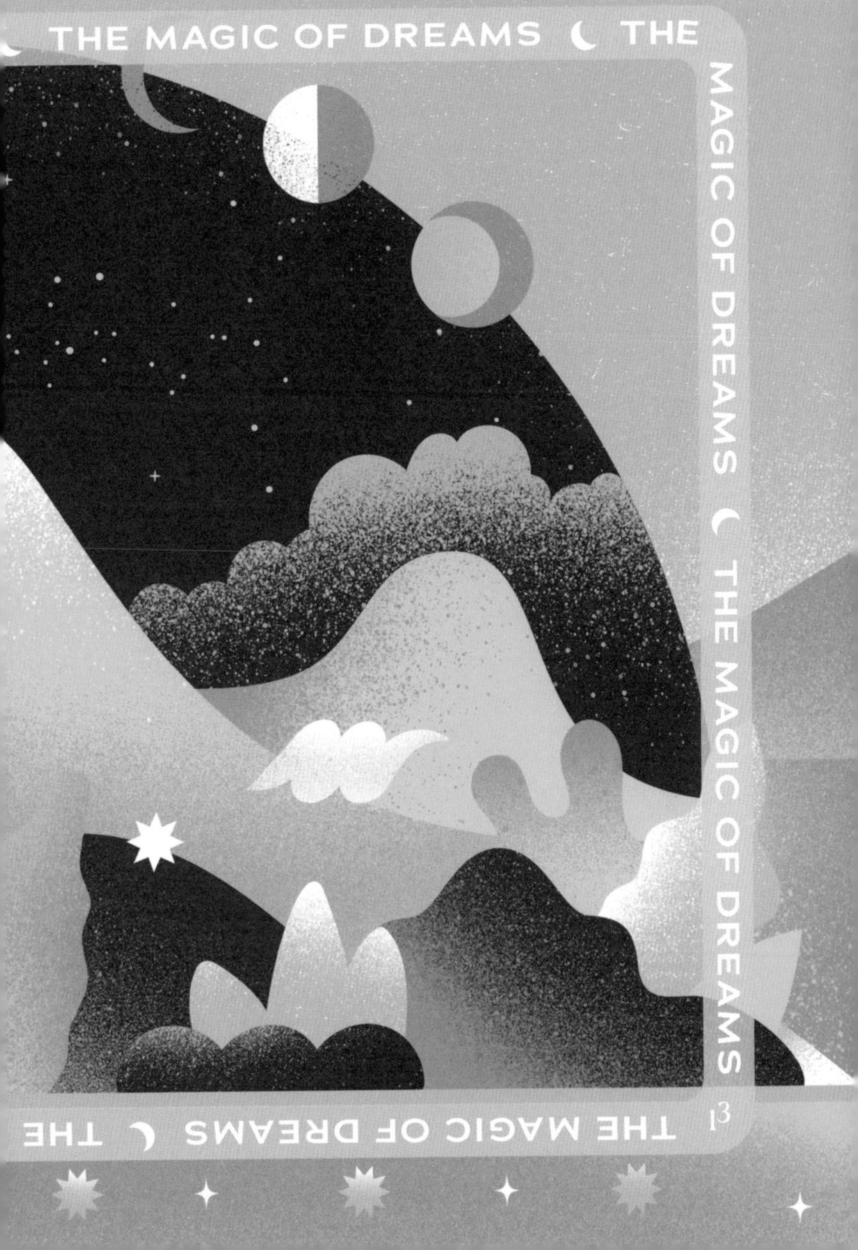
THE MAGIC OF DREAMS THE
THE MAGIC OF DREAMS
THE MAGIC OF DREAMS
THE MAGIC OF DREAMS THE

THE MAGIC OF DREAMS

The Dream Realm

From the peaceful to the exhilarating, and even the downright terrifying, our dreams are as much a source of fascination as they are confusion. But beneath their puzzling exterior lies a wellspring of great personal truth. Creating a living bridge between the unconscious and conscious realms, dreams serve as magical doorways to our deepest selves, bringing our hidden desires, feelings, and fears out of the darkness and up to the surface.

In helping us uncover thoughts and emotions that are below our conscious awareness (the subconscious), as well as suppressed feelings, concealed phobias, and past memories that are buried so deep that we have no awareness of them (the unconscious), dreams ultimately speak to our soul's inherent wisdom, providing powerful opportunities to transform our waking lives.

Whether it's your first time working with dreams or you regularly interpret them, know that you're already an expert. Though you may not feel like it, the power to understand your dreams is an ability that only you possess and have always had. After all, dreams are highly personal in nature. Spun from the fabric of your experiences and woven together by your sleeping mind, dreams are like one-of-a-kind messages cut from the cloth of your subconscious. Your memories, emotions, hopes, fears, perspectives, beliefs, and values are unlike anyone else's and, therefore, they will color your dreams in ways that only you can fully realize. It comes as no surprise, then, that the best person to illuminate the true meaning of your dreams is YOU—the dreamer.

If you're ready to peer beyond the veil of your subconscious and step into the seat of your intuitive wisdom, I invite you to learn about the magic of dreams. In the pages ahead, you'll discover what ancient cultures believed about dreams, modern day dream theories, and how intuitive dream interpretation can enrich your life.

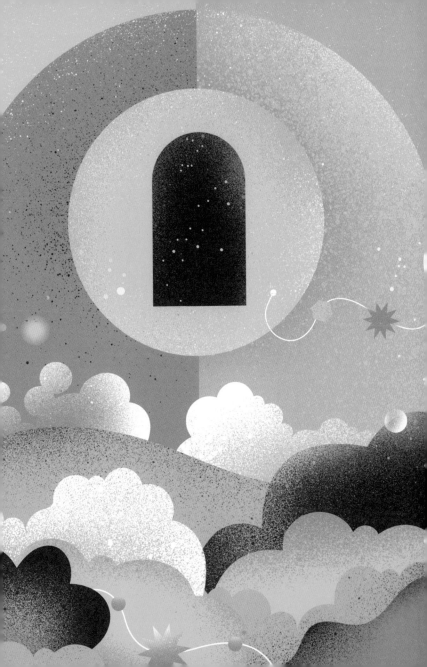

A History of Dreams

If you're wondering why you dream and what your dreams mean, you're not alone. Since the beginning of recorded history, humankind has attempted to answer these age-old questions, producing a trail of interpretations and theories that have spanned across the millennia. From foreshadowing danger to serving as divine messages, dreams have continuously been looked to as a source of guidance in nearly every culture on the planet.

The earliest recorded dream interpretations trace back to ancient Mesopotamia, around 3000 to 4000 BCE, where the Sumerians documented dream symbols and their meanings on clay tablets. During this period, dreams were revered for their spiritual significance and were believed to be sent by the gods, though nightmares were thought to be sent by demons.

In ancient Egypt, dreams were recorded on papyrus as early as 2000 BCE. The Egyptians saw dreams as a way to directly commune with their gods, and believed that those with vivid dreams were gifted with special insight. To strengthen communication with the gods and enhance and summon the dreaming process, they employed a method called incubation, which involved sleeping in a sacred place, such as a temple, or on sanctified "dream beds." This practice became so popular that it was eventually discouraged by temple priests, who instructed citizens to sleep in their own homes before bringing their dreams to special oracles for interpretation.

Throughout the ancient Greek and Roman eras, dreams continued to serve as prophetic signs and played an important role in both public and private life. Considered a tool of divination, dreams were used in a variety of practices, from diagnosing and treating illnesses to shaping military decisions. Dream interpreters even accompanied political leaders into battle. However, writings from Aristotle, a Greek philosopher, and Hippocrates, a Greek physician, were some of the first to suggest that dreams may not have a divine source, asserting that they most likely originate from within the dreamer's own mind.

In ancient China, many believed that a person's soul and spirit left the body while dreaming, transporting them to another dream world each night. They also believed that being suddenly awakened could prevent the soul from returning to the body. Dream symbols were thought to imply auspicious and inauspicious things, depending on the way they were perceived by the dreamer.

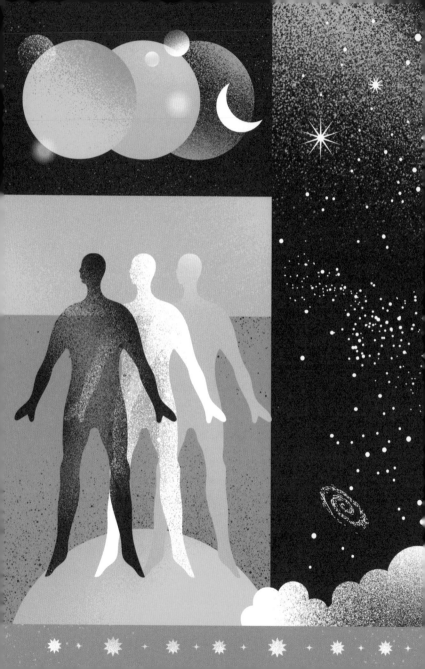

To this day, dreamwork is an integral part of many Indigenous peoples' culture. Though practices vary among tribes, many believe dreams to be an extension of reality. Within the sacred dream dimension, it is thought that we can travel beyond the body and limits of time, visiting different realms, communicating with ancestors and spirit guides, and tapping into a more universal consciousness. Dreaming has also been used by some tribes as a survival tool in predicting the location of game.

Although beliefs about dreams differ from culture to culture, it is evident that these nightly stories have a special significance in our lives. Whether documented on stone, paper, or computer screen, dreams have been celebrated and studied throughout the centuries and around the globe. And though our world has certainly changed since ancient times, the questions and mysteries surrounding dreams have not. Dreams are a part of our individual and collective experiences. They speak to our innate curiosity and never-ending quest for meaning. Ultimately, our desire to decode our dreams to better understand ourselves is a fundamental part of being human, and when we learn to embrace the potential of our dreams, we can tap into the possibilities within.

Dream Theories

While dreams were primarily viewed in a spiritual or supernatural sense throughout ancient times, many modern-day dream theories favor a psychological approach, studying the connection between dreams, the mind, and human behavior. During the nineteenth and twentieth centuries, influential psychoanalysts like Sigmund Freud and Carl Jung concluded that dreams offered insights into the mind's inner workings, shedding light on a person's underlying motivations, deepest desires, and subconscious wishes. Although many different dream theories exist today, the vast majority of them speak to the benefits of dreaming in one form or another. Here are a few of the most widely held beliefs about the role of dreams.

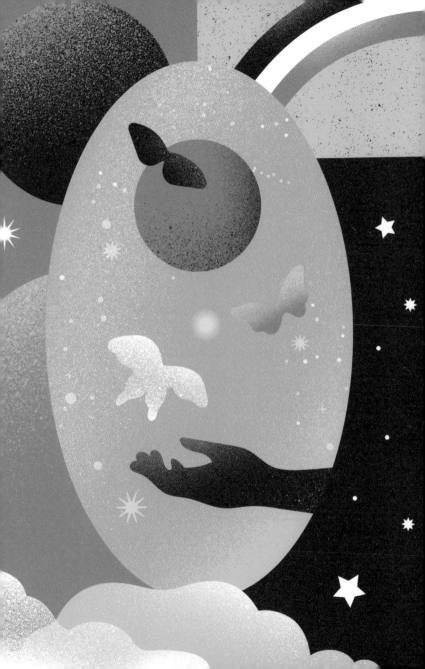

DREAMS PROVIDE A GLIMPSE
INTO OUR SUBCONSCIOUS

In Sigmund Freud's book *The Interpretation of Dreams*, he suggests that dreams are a road map to the unconscious, and that the dream images and symbols we encounter are a reflection of our deepest desires and wishes. Additionally, research from a complementary dream-rebound theory proposes that suppression of a thought tends to result in dreaming about it, supporting the notion that dreams can provide perspective about our unexpressed urges.

DREAMS HELP US PROCESS
EMOTIONS AND MEMORIES

The emotional regulation dream theory holds that dreams are meant to help us cope with and process the emotions that we experience during the day, leading to more balanced and improved moods. Research shows that a strong link exists between REM (rapid eye movement) sleep, emotional memory consolidation, and psychological well-being, suggesting that dreams function as a kind of overnight therapy for emotional events and trauma.

DREAMS PREPARE AND PROTECT
US FROM THREATS

The threat simulation dream theory posits that dreams serve as a type of mental training ground or evolutionary defense mechanism for combating real-world dangers. By simulating social situations and fight-or-flight scenarios, dreams allow us to confront potential threats in a safe environment, leading to better survival strategies and preparedness in waking life.

DREAMS INSPIRE CREATIVITY
AND PROBLEM SOLVING

The creativity theory of dreaming states that dreams help facilitate our creative tendencies and problem-solving abilities by liberating our minds from the constraints of reality. Within the dream realm, our subconscious is free to explore infinite possibilities, allowing us to develop innovative ideas and solutions in the process. Studies show that dreaming supports creative thinking and that many people pull inspiration from their dreams. Deirdre Barrett, an American author and psychologist known for her research on dreams, states that dreaming is simply "thinking in a different biochemical state" and concludes that the mind continues to work on both personal and objective problems while dreaming.

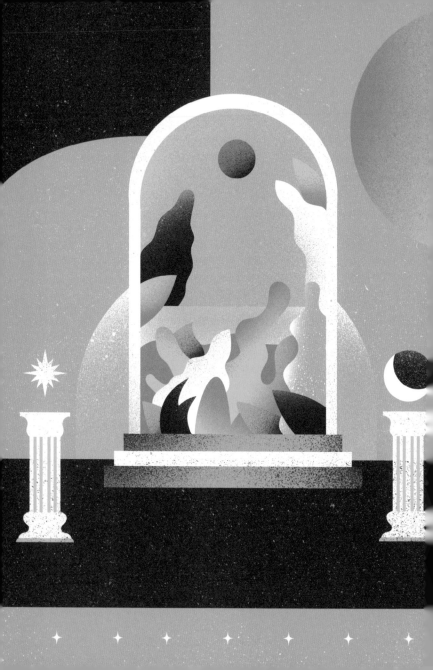

What Happens When We Dream?

Although researchers don't entirely agree on the purpose of dreams, studies show that our bodies undergo a number of physiological changes as we sleep and dream. While sleep has been linked to many health benefits, such as physical restoration, research suggests that deeper sleep stages associated with dreaming may offer a type of mental and emotional replenishment. Here's what we know about what happens during these states and how they affect us.

People tend to think that the brain is "turned off" during sleep, but the unconscious dream state is actually a hotbed of neurological activity. Your brain cycles through four stages of sleep, divided into two phases: non-REM sleep and REM sleep. The first three stages occur during the non-REM sleep phase, in which your brain goes from drowsiness (the transition period between wakefulness and sleep), to light sleep, and finally deep sleep. During non-REM sleep, your heart rate, eye movement, and body temperature decrease. This phase is important for all types of physical restoration, as it allows your body to repair and regenerate tissue, build muscle, and fortify your immune system.

The REM sleep phase is the fourth stage of sleep. It begins about ninety minutes after you fall asleep and repeats every ninety minutes thereafter. The first REM cycle usually lasts about ten minutes and each cycle that follows increases in length, with the final cycle reaching up to as long as one hour. During REM sleep, your eyes move rapidly in different directions and your breathing quickens. Your body also produces cortisol—a chemical responsible for memory consolidation—and glycine, which temporarily paralyzes muscles to prevent you from acting out your dreams in your sleep. Additionally, your heart rate, blood pressure, and brain activity rise to near waking levels, which is why most dreaming and most vivid dreams occur during REM sleep. Although the effects of REM sleep are not entirely known, research suggests that it plays an important role in learning, memory, and mood regulation, as the areas of the brain that support these functions are "turned on" during this phase. Allowing the brain to exercise these important neural connections is thought to be a key component of mental health and overall well-being.

While dream frequency is different for everyone, studies show that people usually dream around four to six times per night, and spend as much as two hours dreaming per night. Some dreams may only last a few seconds, while others can take up to twenty to thirty minutes. During a typical lifetime, it is estimated that the average person spends about twenty-six years sleeping—six of which are spent dreaming! But if dreams are something that happen on a nightly basis, then why is it so difficult to recall them? Dreams are hard to remember primarily because norepinephrine—the brain chemical associated with memory—happens to be at its lowest levels while dreaming. The sleep phase that you wake up from is another big factor. You are far more likely to remember your dreams if you wake up in the REM phase versus a non-REM phase. Since only 20 percent of our total sleep is spent in REM sleep, timing this small window just right can prove tricky.

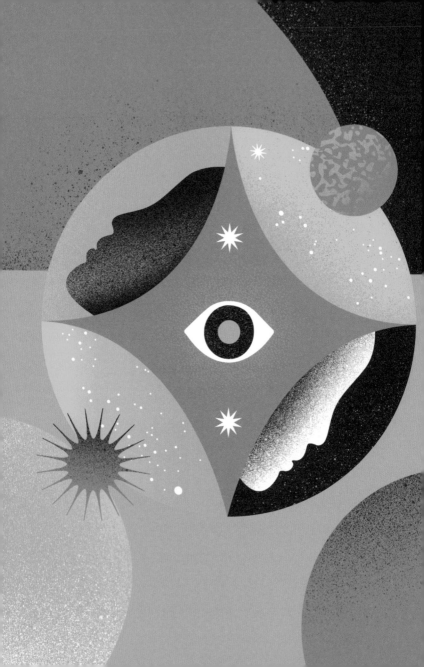

Intuitive Dream Interpretation

Whether dreams carry divine messages, bring omens of the future, or grant insight into the self, the process of interpreting them is highly symbolic. Because dreams communicate through symbols and metaphors, trying to understand their meaning can feel like translating a secret code. However, dream interpretation doesn't have to be overly complicated or cryptic. The truth is, it's as simple as listening to your inner voice.

When it comes to interpreting your dreams, your intuition is your best guide. This is because the magic of dreams lies in discovering what they mean to you personally. Although some symbols can have a universal meaning, such as a clock being equated with time, interpreting dreams is more about exploring your personal connection to the symbol and how it relates to your current life context. Are you anxious about a big deadline, excited for an upcoming event, or thinking about starting a family? A clock can speak to any number of meanings because dream interpretation is almost entirely subjective.

If you've ever consulted an "A to Z" dream dictionary or dream meaning website, then you've likely seen examples of this, as many of them contain a variety of definitions for what a dream symbol could mean. Unfortunately, in most cases, using sources like these only leads to more confusion and frustration. This is because no dream dictionary can tell you what your opinion about something is. This is up to you alone. At the end of the day, your dreams are unique to you, and their answers will be unique to you too.

So how can you transform vague dream symbols and fuzzy metaphors into nuggets of crystal-clear insight? Your intuition holds the key. When you stop trying to fit your specific dream into another person's general expla-nations, and start tuning into your inherent wisdom, the answers you seek will begin to unfold. Like your personal North Star, your intuition is constantly sending you signals from your subconscious. These signals serve to protect you, inspire you, and, ultimately, guide you in the direc-tion that is right for you. That said, learning to intuitively interpret your dreams means you must first learn how to harness your intuition.

THE POWER OF INTUITION

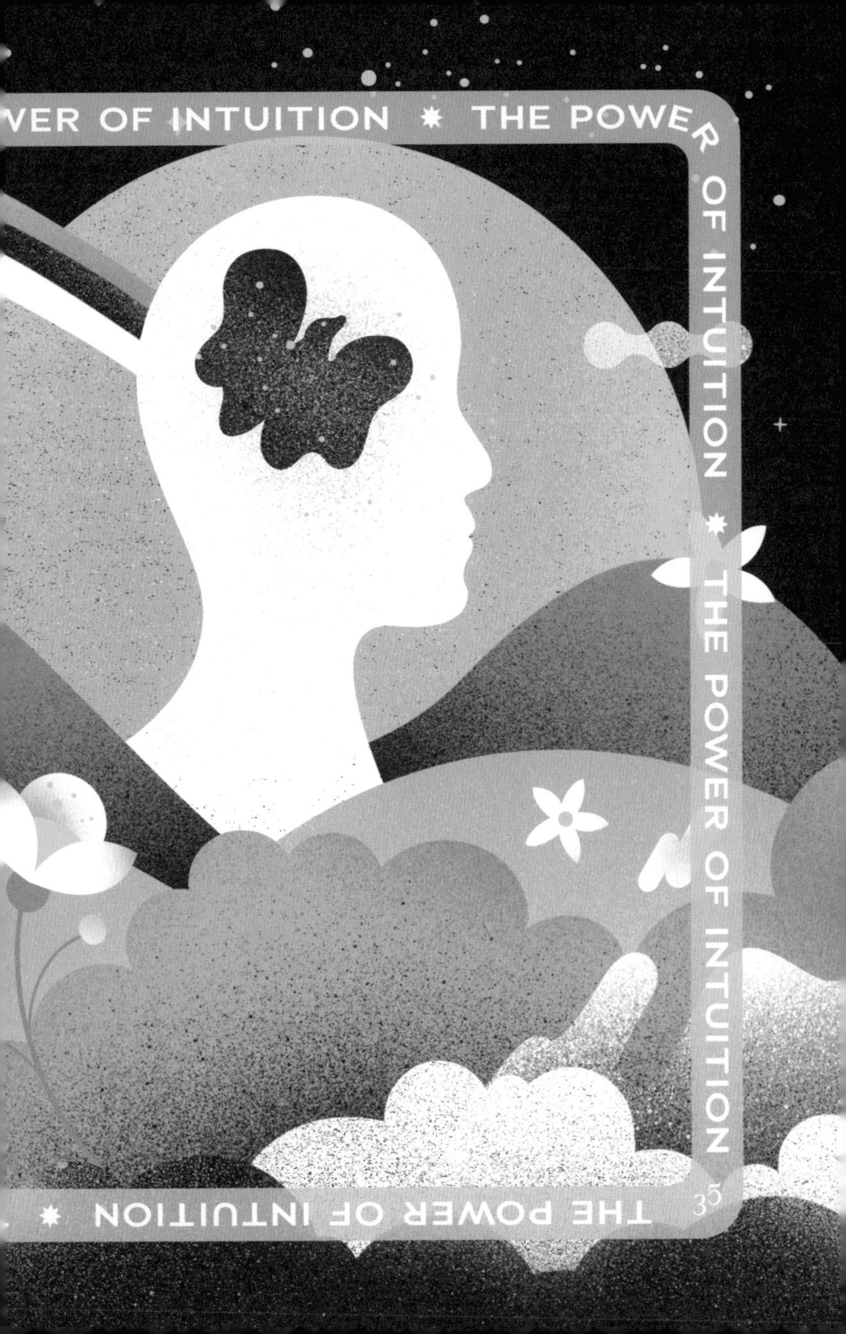
VER OF INTUITION ✸ THE POWER OF INTUITION ✸ THE POWER OF INTUITION
✸ THE POWER OF INTUITION

THE POWER OF INTUITION

What Is Intuition?

Intuition is a feeling, an inkling, a hunch. A sixth sense. Something you just *know*. However you want to describe it, there are instances when conscious reasoning is superseded by a greater gut instinct and immediate understanding. In these moments, you don't need a second opinion or extra time to think things through, because your inner guide already knows the answers. This is the power of intuition.

Flowing from a place of deep, inner resonance, your intuition is the seat of your innate wisdom. It's the voice that suddenly warns you of danger or spurs you to take a leap of faith, despite circumstances that may suggest otherwise. Although these snap judgments may seem to arise without any logical explanation, they tend to leave us with feelings that we simply can't ignore, and usually for good reason. In bringing messages from our subconscious mind to our conscious awareness, our intuition allows us to receive vital information that the rational-thinking mind cannot access. And there's a lot of it.

Studies show that 95 percent of our brain activity happens on a subconscious level, indicating that only 5 percent of our cognitive activity comes from our conscious mind. This means that the large majority of our waking actions—including our decisions, behaviors, and emotions—are being influenced beyond our conscious awareness. Each day, we take in massive amounts of information through our senses, which our brain attempts to process and store at lightning speed. However, there are limits to how much the cognitive mind can handle. Much of this raw material "overflows" into the subconscious mind, forming a pool of past memories and environmental cues that serve to inform our future decisions. So, if something feels amiss, or you notice a subtle shift in perception, know that it's your intuition working behind the scenes, silently pulling from this pool of experiences to signal you a message. Oftentimes, these messages come to us in the form of dreams. Whether you choose to listen to them or not is up to you, but if you do, these messages can alter the course of your life in ways you've never imagined.

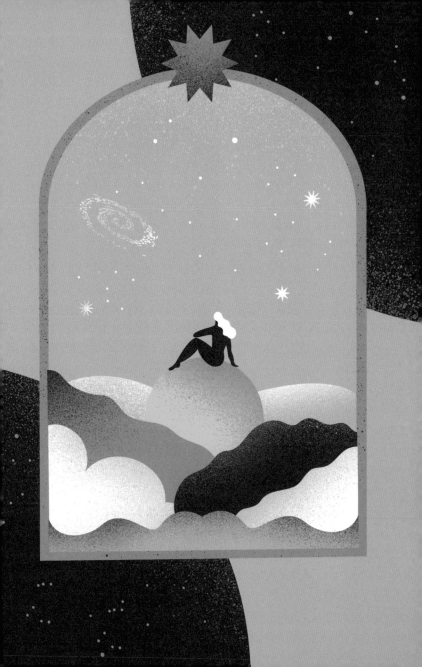

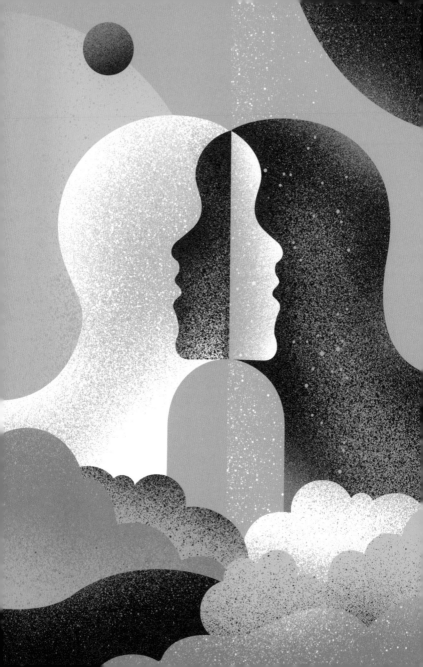

How Your Intuition Speaks to You

You've probably heard phrases like "follow your intuition" or "trust your gut" before, but how can you be certain that what you're feeling is the real deal? Although leaning into your intuition sounds like something that should be second nature, picking up signals from your subconscious requires a certain degree of self-awareness. To better understand this process, think of a radio or TV. These electronic devices transmit information—whether music, pictures, or conversations—through invisible radio waves. Like most subconscious messages, these waves go largely undetected without the proper equipment. In this sense, tapping into your intuition is a lot like tuning into a radio station. In order to hear what's playing, you have to find the right frequency. This involves tuning into a state of active listening and intention. When you dial into your feelings and enter a place of receptivity, you facilitate communication between your subconscious and conscious mind, allowing messages to come through loud and clear.

Your intuition speaks to you through a variety of senses—through something you see, hear, feel, taste, or touch, or via a psychic sixth sense. It can feel subtle at times, and more obvious at others. We all experience our intuition a little differently, though there are a few common signs that may indicate that your intuition is trying to speak to you.

———

YOU FEEL A SENSE OF PEACE OR UNEASE IN YOUR BODY

Many people experience intuition as a physical feeling within the body, particularly the stomach, but these sensations aren't strictly limited to the gut. Ultimately, listening to your intuition is about reading your body as a whole. Some describe their intuition as a general sense of peacefulness or uneasiness, marked by "expansive" or "contractive" feelings. Expansive feelings typically occur when you're in sync with your intuition, while contractive feelings may indicate that something is off. When you scan your body for sensations, pay attention to whether they feel light, open, and energizing (expansive) or heavy, tight, and slow (contractive). The latter may manifest as a sinking feeling in the stomach, tightness in the chest, clenched jaw, headache, or scattered mind.

YOU HAVE MOMENTS OF CLARITY WHEN YOU SLOW DOWN

Your intuitive voice is loudest when your mind is quiet and still. If you've ever had an "aha!" moment in the shower or a sudden epiphany while driving, this could be a sign that your intuition is speaking to you. Activities that help your mind slow down and rest, such as meditation, provide space for your inner feelings to surface. Because most intuitive messages are drowned out by the nonstop noise of the day, it's important to pause every now and then and notice the sensations that arise.

YOU CAN'T SEEM TO SHAKE CERTAIN THOUGHTS AND IDEAS

If you've been consciously ignoring intuitive hints, or missing them by accident, there's a good chance they'll keep showing up in one form or another. Having recurring thoughts and ideas could imply that your intuition is guiding you, so if you notice that your attention keeps slipping in a certain direction, stop to consider why this may be happening. Repeating patterns are your intuition's way of pointing out things you may have overlooked.

YOU FEEL CONFIDENT IN A
DECISION THAT ISN'T RATIONAL

Have you ever felt so confident in a decision, even if it wasn't the most logical choice? Perhaps you decided to quit a secure job, leave a steady relationship, or go back to school. Others may have tried to dissuade you from these choices, but at the end of the day, you knew what was right for you. If you've experienced something similar, this could be a signal from your intuition. Remember, your intuition comes from a place of deep inner knowing, which may sometimes feel at odds with your protective instincts or ego.

YOU HAVE VIVID OR LUCID DREAMS

Your dreams are a gateway to your subconscious. Since sleep quiets the cognitive, rational-thinking mind, intuitive messages can easily work their way into your dreams. If you experience particularly vivid dreams, or lucid dreaming, which occurs when the dreamer is aware that they are dreaming, this may indicate that your intuition is communicating with you.

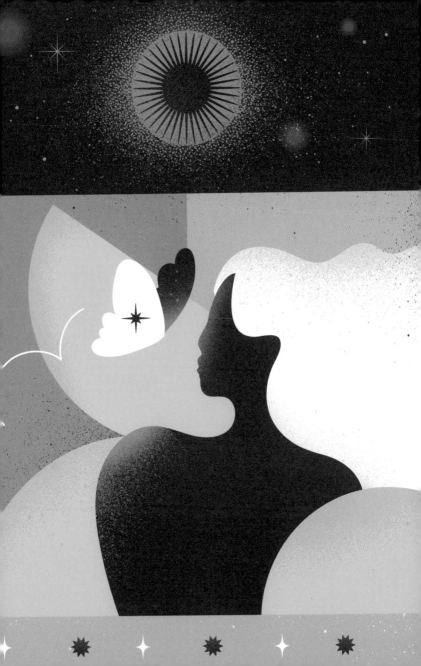

Learning to Trust Your Intuition

Tugging at our consciousness, the invisible strings of our intuition are always there. Quiet, yet implicit, they urge us to go with our gut. Still, placing our trust in this unseen force—especially one that goes against our learned habits and protective instincts—is easier said than done. Not only that, but these intuitive messages are often so subtle that we tend to miss them altogether or suppress them without even realizing it. If intuition is something we're born with, then why do we struggle to use it?

There are a few reasons why trusting our intuitive voice is difficult. Since birth, we've been taught to look outside of ourselves for answers. Society has constantly pushed the belief that what we seek—whether validation, truth, permission, or love—can only be gained through external sources. Instead of relying on our own perceptions and intuitions, we are told to discount them in favor of what family members, authority figures, or religious or academic institutions deem meaningful. Now, this isn't to say that outside sources can't be useful. In fact, there are plenty of situations in which seeking a second opinion is not only helpful but recommended. However, when we begin to rely too heavily on the outer world for answers, we run the risk of diluting our own inner wisdom.

Learning to trust your intuitive voice is the ultimate act of trusting yourself, but there are a few common road-blocks that you may encounter during the process. Before you embark on your intuitive journey, take note of these potential pitfalls so that you can easily identify and resolve them, should they occur.

————

EXTERNAL OPINIONS

A major part of cultivating your intuition is listening to yourself. If you tend to give others' opinions more weight than your own, or find that your decisions hinge upon another's approval, you may end up making choices that aren't in alignment with your highest good. The truth is, many people throughout your life will have ideas about what is best for you. Some may be well intentioned, while others will have their own interests in mind. Regardless, no one can speak to what you actually feel in your gut. You alone have to make the call.

OVERTHINKING

When left unchecked, the cognitive, rational-thinking mind is one of the largest obstacles to embracing your intuition. Concerned with fact rather than feeling, the rational-thinking mind is designed to follow what makes sense. So while the ability to analyze your options and run through different mental scenarios may work to your advantage most of the time, it can also cause you to overthink or second-guess your choices. Constantly weighing the pros and cons of a situation can even leave you in a state of "analysis paralysis," a dizzying cycle of overthinking that makes you unable to move forward.

THE EGO

Your ego can generally be described as your mind's constructed identity, or who you think you are. This false sense of self creates a powerful illusion that not only hinders the intuitive process but also blocks you from your full potential. Because the ego is rooted in fear, listening to its demands can keep you trapped in a cycle of negative thoughts and limiting beliefs (e.g., thinking "I'm not good enough," or "I'm not smart enough").

LACK OF REST

A jam-packed schedule leaves little room for intuitive guidance to slip through. If you've been running yourself ragged and can never seem to catch your breath, it's going to be hard to notice when your intuition is speaking to you. Most people experience intuitive hits during quiet periods of alone time or self-reflection, so a busy calendar could mean that you've been brushing these inklings to the wayside.

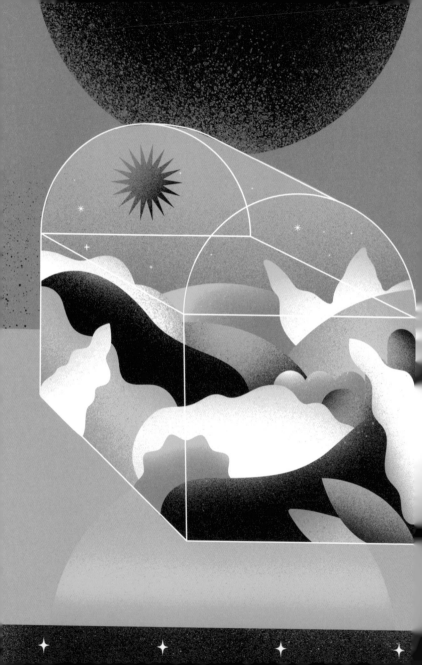

How to Cultivate Your Intuition

If you've encountered some intuitive roadblocks, or are still uncertain about how to tap into your intuition, don't fret! Even those who have been out of touch with their intuition their whole lives can learn to summon its wisdom. Your intuition operates on such a deeply instinctual level that you can access it anytime, though using it intentionally requires practice and patience. You can think of your intuition as a muscle to strengthen. The more deliberately you train it and consistently use it, the more powerful it will become.

To cultivate your intuition, consider the following practices. Keep in mind that this process is a lifelong journey—one that will lead you back through these steps time and time again. Be compassionate with yourself as you develop these skills and take the time you need to hone them. The more you work on harnessing your intuition, the more easily you'll be able to apply it to dream interpretation.

TRUST IN THE PROCESS

Working with your intuition isn't always a clear-cut process. It can feel messy and confusing, especially at first. What's important to remember during these initial stages is that not everything is going to make sense. Intuition, by nature, is not logical or rational, so refrain from treating it like a puzzle. Your intuition doesn't need to be "fixed" or "solved." If you trust in the process, believe in your intuition, and have faith in yourself, the answers will come.

SCAN YOUR BODY FOR SENSATIONS

Your intuition is constantly communicating with you via the senses, so performing a head-to-toe body scan is one of the easiest ways to check in. Find a quiet space to meditate, close your eyes, and begin to scan through your body for sensations. Start at the top of your head and work your way down to your toes, spending a few minutes in each area. Noticing the physical sensations that arise (e.g., tingling, warmth, soreness, tension, etc.) can clue you in to your emotional state and allow you to be more present with your feelings.

SLOW DOWN YOUR MIND

Surrendering the cognitive, rational-thinking mind is one of the biggest challenges to activating your intuition, so it's important to create opportunities for your brain to rest. When you practice slowing down, both mentally and physically, you'll be better able to acknowledge and process the messages that you receive. Set aside time for activities that get you out of your head and into your body, such as yoga, meditation, or mindful breathing exercises.

BE PATIENT

Intuition isn't something that you can force or rush, so be patient when seeking answers. Fear can create a false sense of urgency that muddles intuitive messages, so as tempting as it may be to look outside yourself for answers, try to let things unfold at their natural pace. Answers may not emerge overnight, but by remaining open and receptive to your intuition, you'll be able to perceive situations more clearly.

FOCUS ON YOUR NEEDS

Listening to your intuition means asking yourself, "What do I need right now? What is important for me in this moment?" As you answer these questions, keep the focus on you. This is a time to honor your innermost feelings and desires rather than catering to what other people want. That said, if you notice your attention drifting back to others' opinions or expectations, acknowledge that they are not a part of your truth and gently set them aside.

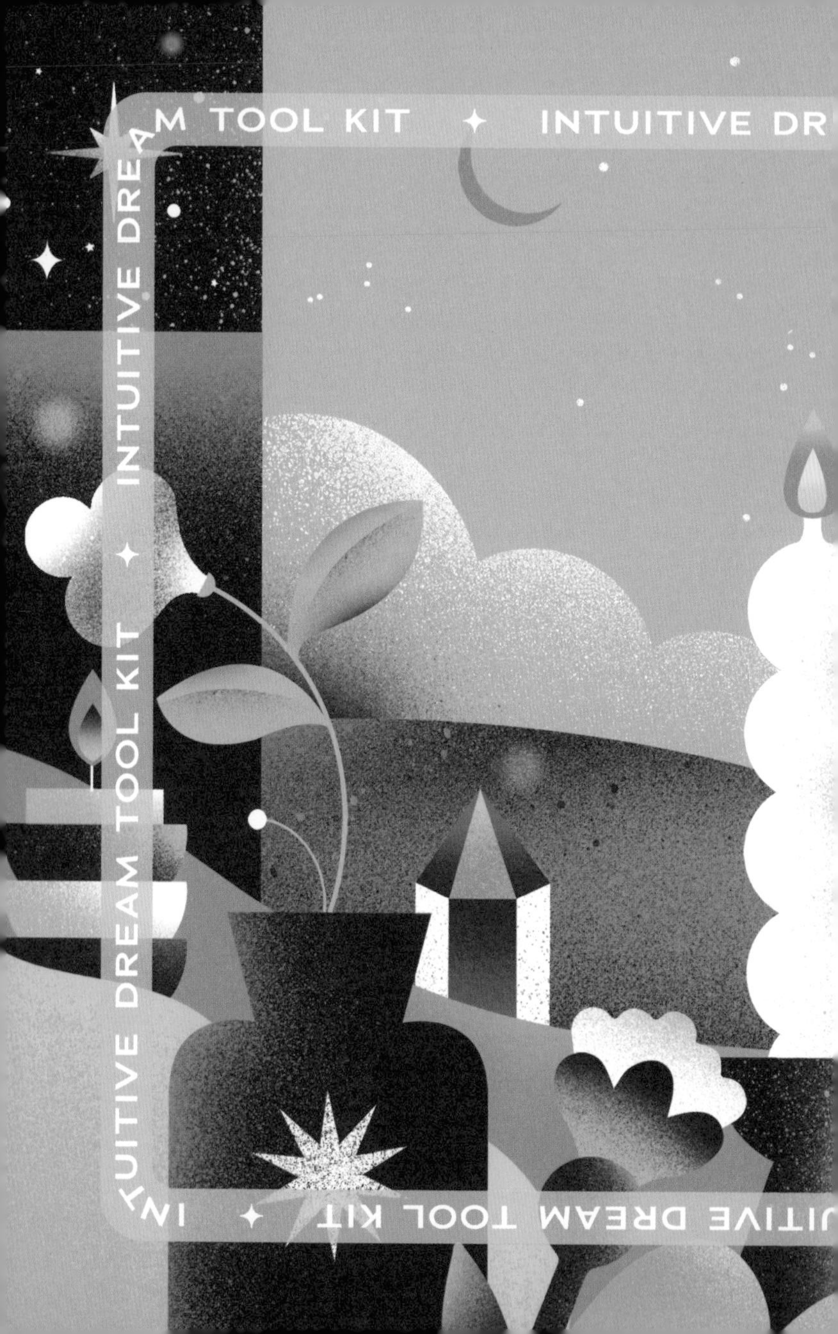

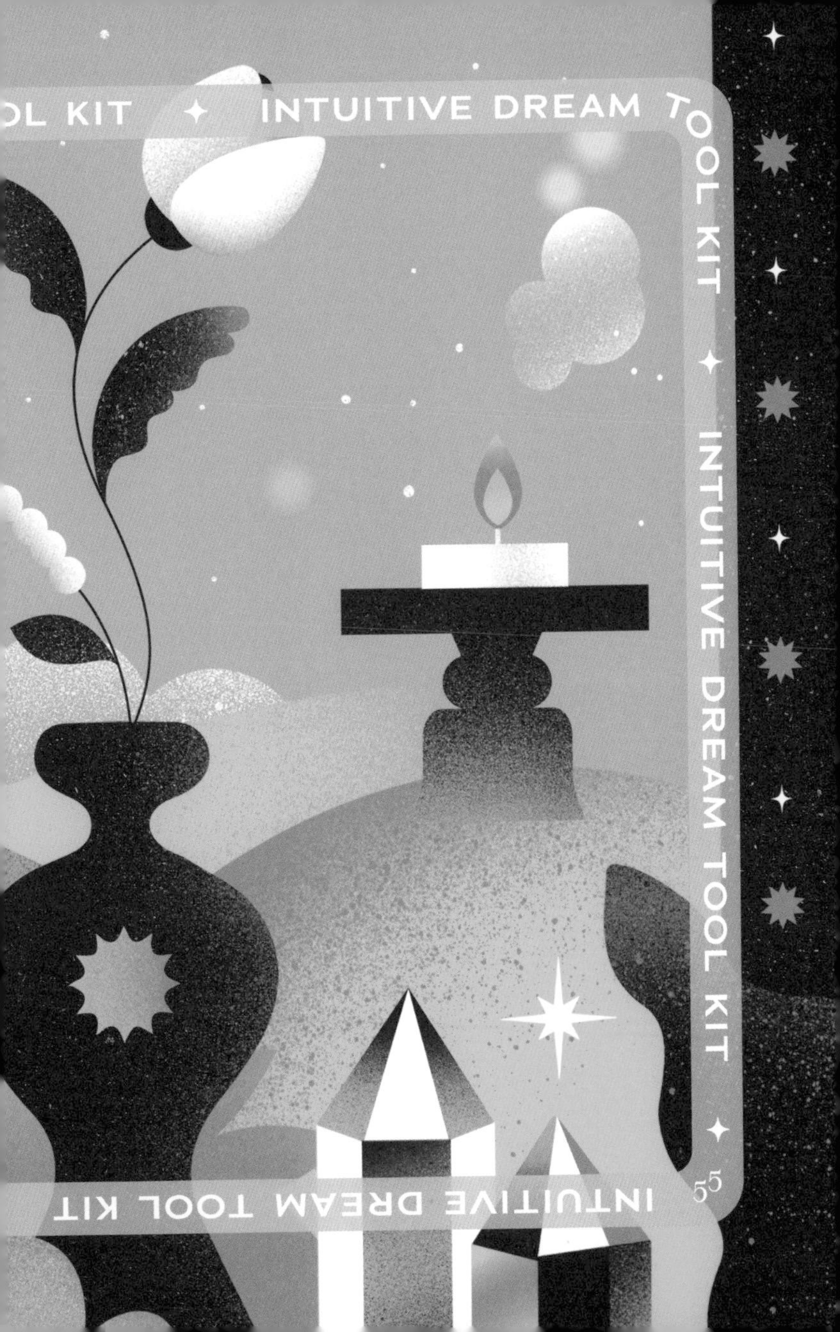
INTUITIVE DREAM TOOL KIT

INTUITIVE DREAM TOOL KIT

Supporting Your Dream Experience

Welcome to your go-to resource for working with dreams. The Intuitive Dream Tool Kit features a collection of practices, tools, and gentle techniques designed to energetically support dreamers of any experience level, day or night. In this section, you'll find wellness tips, herbs, crystals, and affirmations to help deepen your connection to your dreams and intuition and enhance your quality of sleep. We've divided the tool kit into two parts, Before Sleep and After Waking, which focus on evening and morning rituals, respectively. Use those in Before Sleep to promote relaxation and attract good dreams at night, and those in After Waking to elevate your dream awareness and intuition during the day.

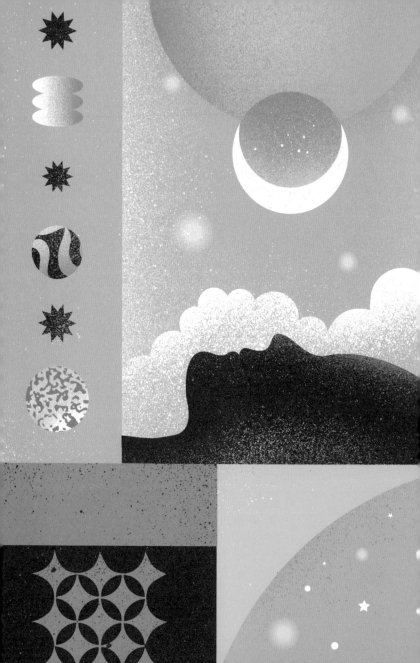

Before Sleep

Wellness Tips

While there is no right or wrong way to dream, there are a few practices that can set you up for a successful night of sleep that invites more dream opportunities. Here are a few ways to improve your overall sleep quality and make the most of your dream experience.

CREATE A COMFORTABLE ENVIRONMENT

Creating a relaxing and comfortable environment is essential not only for falling asleep quickly, but also for staying asleep. Review your current bedroom setup and consider these points when designing your sleep space:

> Use a high-quality mattress and pillow: Your mattress is the foundation of your sleep environment. A quality mattress will ensure that your spine is supported and aligned, and a good pillow will do the same for your

head and neck. If aches and pains frequently keep you up at night, it may be time to swap out these items. It is recommended that mattresses be replaced every seven to ten years.

> **Choose season-appropriate bedding:**
  Switching out your sheets and blankets to suit your location's climate can help with temperature regulation and save you money in the long run. For warmer months, select light and breathable fabrics to wick away moisture and keep you cool, such as silk, satin, bamboo, linen, or cotton. For colder months, use heavier fabrics with heat-insulating qualities, such as cotton fleece, flannel, wool, cashmere, or polyester. These guidelines apply to sleepwear too!

> **Set an agreeable temperature:** Being too hot or too cold can affect your ability to sleep through the night. Pick an agreeable temperature that allows you to sleep without disruption. Although the ideal temperature varies by person, most research shows that sleeping in a cooler room—around 65 degrees Fahrenheit (18 degrees Celsius)—can improve sleep.

KEEP DISTRACTIONS
TO A MINIMUM

A distraction-free space makes for a better sleep experience. By limiting light, noise, and notifications throughout the night, you'll be able to reduce fragmented sleep cycles and improve rest.

> **Avoid light disruption:** Excess light exposure compromises your body's ability to sleep. To reduce light exposure, turn down your lights and put away your electronic devices. For total darkness, invest in blackout curtains or wear an eye mask.

> **Reduce noise:** Loud noises can jolt you awake at night, but even the ones that don't wake you up can subconsciously affect your sleep patterns by reducing the time you spend in deeper sleep stages, such as slow wave and REM sleep. To promote peace and quiet in the bedroom, add soft surfaces like rugs and curtains to absorb and dampen noise, and insulate your windows to seal off sounds from outside. If you can't eliminate nearby sources of noise, consider using a white noise machine to drown out competing sounds, or try wearing earplugs.

> Disconnect from your devices: The blue light emitted from phone screens and computers has been shown to disrupt circadian rhythms by suppressing the body's release of melatonin—a hormone that makes us feel drowsy. Limit your time on these devices by switching them to Do Not Disturb mode after work, or putting them away completely at least thirty minutes before bed.

FINE-TUNE YOUR SLEEP SCHEDULE

Harnessing the full benefits of sleep means making it a priority. By implementing conscious strategies to optimize your sleep, you'll be able to take control of your daily sleep schedule in powerful and effective ways.

> Pay attention to your circadian rhythm: Syncing your sleep schedule to your body's natural sleep-wake cycle, or circadian rhythm, can positively impact sleep. To do so, notice when you naturally start to feel sleepy in the evening, and what time you wake up at without an alarm clock. Going to bed and waking up around these times will complement your natural energy levels and make it easier to be consistent. Be mindful of

any habits that can throw your schedule off track, such as staying on your phone late at night, which may unintentionally push back your bedtime.

> **Budget time for sleep:** Research suggests that healthy adults need between seven and nine hours of sleep each night. When planning your day, be sure to factor in ample sleep time. Don't compromise it by overscheduling yourself.

> **Set consistent sleep and wake times:** Going to bed at the same time each night and getting up at the same time each morning helps regulate your body's internal clock. To stay on track, set evening reminders on your phone for when it's time to start winding down.

> **Make changes gradually:** If your sleep schedule has gotten derailed, there's no need for a giant overhaul. The best way to change your sleep schedule is to make small, incremental adjustments over time (with a maximum difference of one to two hours per night) so that your body can slowly adapt. By making these gradual shifts, you'll be able to reach your target time at a sustainable pace and follow your new schedule with ease.

Herbs

Relaxation is vital to any interpretation practice, as it forms the foundation of rest. Without relaxation, it can be incredibly difficult to fall asleep or reach deeper sleep stages, such as REM sleep, when most dreams occur. Luckily, there are a number of herbal allies that can be used to soothe the mind, dissolve stress, and support dreamwork.

FOR PROMOTING DREAMS

Mugwort

A member of the daisy family, mugwort is considered a common weed, but its applications are extensive. It's been used in everything from food to dyes to insect repellent, and boasts a number of health benefits, such as calming nerves, promoting digestion, and regulating menstrual cycles. Mugwort is an exceptional tool for dreamwork and divination, as it has been used throughout the centuries to deepen meditation, induce vivid dreams, and help people access their intuitive guidance. It also shares a strong connection to lunar energy.

Usage tips: To encourage memorable dreams, drink a cup of mugwort tea before bed, or use its dried leaves to create a dream sachet. A dream sachet is a small cloth bag filled with herbs, flowers, or other aromatic ingredients that is placed under a pillow to promote dreams. Yours can be as simple as stuffing an old sock or you can sew one from the material of your choosing. Combine it with dried lavender for relaxation and protection within dreams. Note: Those allergic to ragweed should avoid using mugwort.

FOR INTUITIVE ASCENSION

Blue Lotus

Blue lotus assists in connecting you to higher states of consciousness and expanding awareness of the dream state. Equal parts sedative and stimulant, it provides a mild sense of tranquility and euphoria and possesses a gentle, uplifting effect. In modern Western herbalism, blue lotus is considered an antidepressant, antioxidant, aphrodisiac, antispasmodic, and anti-inflammatory herb. Working with blue lotus before bed can aid your transition into the lucid dream state by pleasantly opening up your sensory and intuitive capacities.

Usage tips: To strengthen awareness of your dreams, consume a cup of blue lotus tea before bedtime. Tea is the most traditional way to experience this herb, though blue lotus petals can be burned as incense, smoked ceremonially, or infused into oil. To create a pain-relieving body massage oil, add the desired amount of dried petals to your carrier oil of choice, such as almond oil, and let the mixture steep for two to six weeks, shaking daily. Strain out the petals before use.

FOR ENHANCING RELAXATION

Passionflower

Visually stunning passion-flower is a climbing vine that is used in a number of herbal medicines and supplements. Known for easing stress, tension, and anxiety, it provides support to the nervous system by promoting a state of relaxation, which helps facilitate dreams. Use it to unwind at the end of the day or soothe an unsettled stomach.

Usage tips: If restless thoughts keep you up at night, sip a cup of passionflower tea right before bed. For best results, drink one cup of tea every night for at least seven days to feel the full effects. Incorporating an affirmation for calming or release, such as "I embrace inner peace" or "I release today," can provide further support to your dreams by clear-ing away any lingering energetic attachments. Repeat the affirmation aloud before you take your first sip.

✦ INTUITIVE DREAM TOOL KIT ✦

FOR SUPPORTING DEEP SLEEP

Valerian Root

Often referred to as "nature's Valium," valerian root contains powerful soothing and sleep-enhancing properties. Like passionflower, it helps reduce anxiety and promote relaxation, but with the added benefit of supporting deep sleep. Research suggests that taking valerian root may not only help you fall asleep faster but also achieve deep sleep more quickly. Its insomnia-relieving effects are seemingly caused by boosting the level of gamma-aminobutyric acid (GABA) in the brain, which produces a calming effect that allows for better sleep.

Usage tips: Valerian root can be taken as a capsule, tablet, liquid extract, or tea. It is recommended that it be taken thirty minutes to two hours before sleep. Dried valerian can be added to a dream sachet or pillow to improve sleep quality and ward off nightmares. For protection at home, sprinkle some of its powder around your front door.

Crystals

Crystals can improve sleep quality and promote peaceful dreams by bringing the mind and body to a state of quiet relaxation before bed. Though there are countless crystals to choose from in the mineral kingdom, there are a few whose soothing and sleep-enhancing qualities are particularly well suited for dreamwork.

FOR ENCOURAGING DEEP SLEEP

Amethyst

When it comes to getting a good night's sleep, there is no better stone than amethyst. Known for its soothing and serene vibrations, amethyst calms the mind and induces a peaceful, meditative state, making it an ideal companion for drifting off to sleep. Not only that, but its protective and purifying properties improve overall sleep quality by warding off nightmares and reducing insomnia. If you struggle with both falling and staying asleep, working with amethyst can deliver the disruption-free rest you've been waiting for.

Mini ritual: Meditate with this stone over your third eye chakra (located in the center of the forehead, between the brows) before bed to quiet the cognitive mind and open yourself to your inner wisdom. After you've taken a few minutes to align with its calming frequency, place the stone underneath your pillow or on a nightstand to promote deep sleep. Since amethyst has a high vibration, those who are sensitive to crystals may benefit from using gentler alternatives, such as moonstone or selenite.

FOR RELIEVING STRESS AND ANXIETY

Lepidolite

Does the stress of the day keep you up at night? Luckily, frayed nerves are no match for lepidolite. Considered one of the best crystals for sleep problems, lepidolite contains lithium, which is used to treat mood swings and depression, giving it a natural tranquilizing effect. If anger, fear, or anxiety is pushing you to emotional extremes, use this stone to restore your sense of balance and gently return back to center.

Mini ritual: Hold this stone in your hand and breathe deeply as you slowly scan your body from head to toe, noticing any areas of tension or tightness. If you encounter any, focus on relaxing the muscles in that area before moving on to the next until all pressure points have been dissolved. If you are using a tumbled piece of lepidolite, or "worry stone," gently rub the stone between your thumb and forefinger to gradually diffuse negativity. Tumbled lepidolite can be placed under your pillow, though rough types are more delicate and should be kept out of the bed.

✦ INTUITIVE DREAM TOOL KIT ✦

FOR ATTRACTING CLEAR MESSAGES

Indigo Gabbro

Strengthening the link between the physical and spiritual realms, indigo gabbro helps attract and capture valuable insights within dreams. This stone is unique in that it serves as a grounded bridge to higher consciousness, opening you to spiritual contact while helping retain its lessons. If you seek to uncover the shadowy aspects of your dreams, this stone will unveil any deeply rooted issues that have been hiding beneath the surface.

Mini ritual: Hold this stone in your hand before you go to bed and say aloud three times, "I attract clear messages into my dreams." Place the stone on top of a dream journal or notebook next to your bed. Keeping these items nearby will encourage you to immediately jot down your dreams upon waking, while the illuminating effects of indigo gabbro help shed light on their hidden meaning.

FOR PROTECTION WHILE DREAMING

Black Tourmaline

A must-have for journeying within dreams, black tourmaline provides energetic protection as you sleep. Its grounding properties form an effective shield against psychic attacks, bad dreams, and all types of negativity. Due to its association with the root chakra, this stone can be used to improve your sense of security, safety, and stability as you actively explore your subconscious.

Mini ritual: Meditate with this stone in your hand before bed. After one to two minutes, repeat aloud the phrase, "I am always safe and protected in my dreams," and then place the crystal under your pillow or on your nightstand. For added protection, pair a few pieces of black tourmaline with selenite to create a powerful crystal grid near your bed. This will not only shield you from unwanted influences in your dreams but also keep the energy of your sacred space continually refreshed.

Affirmations

Incorporating positive affirmations into your evening rituals can enhance your dreams by easing you into a state of rest and receptivity. Whether you need help connecting to your intuition or releasing restless thoughts, affirmations offer a way to consciously harness and direct your energy. You can practice these affirmations by simply stating them aloud before bed or while setting an intention with a crystal. Though this may seem like a small act, regularly using affirmations can help deepen your awareness of your dreams and their insights. To start, repeat one of the following every night, and if/when you feel ready, use your intuition to write your own.

FOR INSIGHTFUL DREAMS

> I open myself to the divine wisdom of my dreams and the unlimited potential of my imagination.

> My dreams always have the answers I am looking for. I listen carefully for their messages.

> Tonight, I ask for dreams that will bring healing, renewal, and welcome changes to my life.

> The more I listen to my dreams, the more I learn, understand, and appreciate about myself.

> My dreams are a gateway to embracing my inner magic, truth, and power.

> Tonight, my dreams will be vivid, clear, and insightful. The messages I need will be easy to recall in the morning.

> In my dreams, I awaken to my true self and embrace all parts of my being.

FOR PEACEFUL SLEEP

> My mind and body are a sanctuary for rest.

> Inner peace is my priority.

> Tonight I ask for a calming dream that brings me peace and serenity.

> With each breath, I melt away the stress of the day.

> When I quiet my mind, I fall asleep quickly and easily.

> I am always safe and protected as I sleep and dream.

> Tomorrow I will wake up feeling recharged, rested, and fully refreshed.

FOR INTUITIVE GUIDANCE

> When my body speaks to me, I choose to listen.

> I honor the transformative power of my heart's intuition.

> I surrender to the illuminating currents of my subconscious.

> I trust my dreams to show me exactly what I need to see.

> I am an open and clear channel for divine guidance.

> I recognize the Source within and the wisdom I carry.

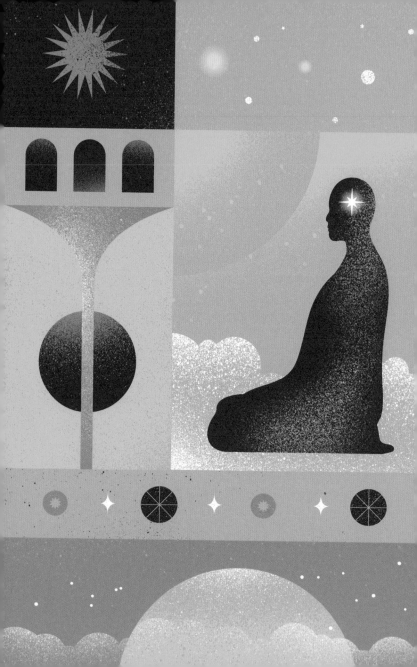

After Waking

Wellness Tips

While your evening routine can have a significant impact on the quality of your sleep and dreams, the same can be said about your daytime habits. To reap the full benefits of your dreams, be mindful of your actions and behaviors during waking hours and how they affect rest, dream recall, and mental clarity.

START YOUR MORNING OFF RIGHT

When and how you wake up in the morning has a direct influence on your ability to recall your dreams, as well as your mood. To facilitate a seamless transition between dreams and wakefulness, consider the following practices.

> **Don't jump out of bed:** When you first wake up, don't move around or open your eyes. Quiet any alarms without looking at devices. These first few moments are crucial for

gathering details from your dreams, which can easily slip away if you start running through your notifications or to-do list. Use this time to drift along your subconscious and bask in any post-dream reflections.

> **Skip the snooze button:** Repeatedly hitting snooze in the morning can throw off your body's waking routine and leave you feeling drowsy for the rest of the day. This fuzzy-headed or groggy sensation is what sleep experts call "sleep inertia," which can last for hours after you wake.

> **Keep it regular:** Waking up at the same time each morning establishes healthy sleep patterns that support your circadian rhythm. Maintaining a steady sleep schedule also helps keep REM periods stable, which is when most dreams occur.

> **Establish a morning routine:** Sticking to a morning routine can help you begin your day with focus and intention. Instead of rushing to work, carve out some extra time in the morning to reground into your physical body and reconnect to your purpose. This can be as simple as light stretches, affirmations, or enjoying a cup of your favorite tea.

CULTIVATE PRO-SLEEP
HABITS DURING THE DAY

Some of your daily habits may be contributing to insomnia and other sleep-related issues. Make sure you are cultivating pro-sleep habits during the day to ensure high-quality sleep at night. Even small adjustments can make a big difference.

> Let the light in: Once you've fully woken up and recorded your dreams, get out in the daylight as soon as possible. Though light exposure at night can throw off your body's internal clock, studies show that morning light exposure results in greater alertness and helps maintain healthy sleep patterns. For best results, get direct sunlight within an hour of waking for a minimum of thirty minutes. Always use sunscreen to protect your skin. It will not impede the process.

> Move your body: Active days make for restful nights. Find time to exercise during the day and get your heart rate up for at least twenty minutes or more to promote longer sleeping times. Avoid working out within two to three hours of bedtime if possible, as this may make it more difficult to fall asleep.

> **Nap responsibly:** Though it may be tempting to squeeze in some extra shut-eye, napping for too long or too late in the day can affect your ability to sleep well at night. Studies show that napping after 3 p.m. can disrupt your natural sleep schedule. Avoid naps if possible, but if you can't, limit them to the early afternoon, for a length of twenty minutes, as this duration is enough to provide restorative sleep.

> **Limit caffeine and alcohol:** Consuming caffeine can make it difficult to fall asleep, due to its stimulating effects, which can last for up to twelve hours. Alcohol, on the other hand, can induce drowsiness due to its sedative properties, but makes it difficult to reach deeper, restorative sleep stages. Be mindful of using either, especially later in the day.

Herbs

Greet the day with clarity and focus by incorporating the following plants and herbs into your morning ritual or during your dream journaling practice. In addition to their many health benefits, these herbs carry a number of spiritual and energetic associations that enhance dream recall and introspection. Use them whenever you need energetic support as you interpret your dreams.

FOR SHAKING OFF GROGGINESS

Lemongrass

Quiet unnecessary mental chatter and instill focus with lemongrass. Lemongrass boasts a variety of physical and spiritual benefits, along with antioxidant, antimicrobial, and anti-inflammatory properties. Featuring a bright, lemony aroma and citrus flavor, lemongrass contains rejuvenating notes that are wonderful for shaking off post-sleep sluggishness and fostering a sense of openness. The uplifting and purifying nature of lemongrass also works to remove distractions from the environment while shedding light on hidden issues.

Usage tips: Meditate with a cup of lemongrass tea after you've recorded your dreams to invigorate and awaken the senses. If you feel your attention drifting away from the interpretation process, spritz a lemongrass spray throughout your sacred space to center your mind and recall your dreams clearly. Lemongrass can also be used to create an all-natural, multipurpose cleaner that can physically and energetically purify your home. Cut up three stalks of lemongrass and two limes (remove peels) into smaller pieces, then add to a clean jar with eight ounces of distilled white vinegar. Seal the jar and let it infuse for two weeks, shaking every few days. Strain out the lemongrass and lime. Use within six months.

FOR BOOSTING MEMORY

Rosemary

An abundant source of antioxidants and anti-inflammatory compounds, rosemary is a fragrant herb with a unique woodsy flavor that is minty, peppery, and piney. Considered a cognitive stimulant, rosemary has been linked to memory for hundreds of years and is said to enhance memory retention and mental alertness. Due to its purifying properties, it can also be used to remove energetic blockages from a person or space.

Usage tips: To dissolve mental blocks and boost memory, use this herb in smoke cleansing. Light a sprig of rosemary and carefully fan its smoke around the room, focusing on corners (where stale energy tends to accumulate). Once you've covered the entire space, place the sprig in a nonflammable bowl to extinguish on its own, then open a window to allow old energy to exit. *Note: Always exercise caution when handling flammable materials indoors. Never leave lit objects unattended. If you are sensitive to smoke, try using rosemary essential oil instead. Apply a couple of drops to your neck or wrist, or use in a diffuser for a burst of mental clarity.*

FOR RAISING SELF-AWARENESS

Nettle

Packed with nutrient-rich vitamins and minerals, nettle provides nourishment to the entire body while regulating hormones and stress. This plant is special in that it affects each person intuitively, picking up on your specific energetic needs. If you need energy, it'll give you energy. If you need to relax, it'll help you do just that. Whatever the case, nettle shines a light on any uncomfortable sensations or feelings outside of your awareness so that they can be addressed.

Usage tips: Fresh nettle leaves should not be eaten, as contact with their barbs can cause irritation (hence the name, "stinging nettles"). However, processed and dried nettles are perfectly safe to use and can be added to teas, soups, and smoothies. If your dreams stir up challenging emotions or experiences, use nettle to sit with your feelings and work through their meaning.

FOR IMPROVING CLARITY

Peppermint

Peppermint is regarded as one of the world's oldest medicines. It has analgesic, astringent, decongestant, antimicrobial, and antiseptic properties, which have been used to treat everything from indigestion to menstrual cramps. Known for its strong cooling effect, peppermint is both relaxing and stimulating, allowing you to interpret your dreams calmly and clearly. Due to its association with the throat chakra, peppermint also encourages communication between the mind and body, helping you tap into your inner voice.

Usage tips: Dry out a few peppermint leaves and press them into the pages of your dream journal, or store them in a small pouch next to your bed. Keeping peppermint in close proximity will encourage a fresh perspective during interpretation and cut through any distracting thoughts. Drinking peppermint tea or using peppermint essential oil can also provide similar effects.

Crystals

Crystals can promote clarity, focus, and introspection. Here we've included crystals that will help you retrieve and retain insights from your dreams while awake. Meditating with these stones before interpreting your dreams will allow you to ground into your physical body while activating your intuition, making you more receptive to messages from your subconscious.

FOR RECALLING DREAMS

Herkimer Diamond

Commonly referred to as "desert diamond," Herkimer diamond is actually a special variety of double-terminated quartz. Featuring exceptional clarity and brightness, this stone boasts an incredibly pure vibration and is said to be the most powerful of all quartz crystals. A must-have for dream recall, this stone will allow you to access dream consciousness while awake, deepen memory and concentration, and provide grounding and clarity after intense spiritual work. It can also support you in receiving guidance from higher dimensions, retrieving past-life information, and lucid dreaming.

Usage tips: If you're struggling to remember your dreams, use this stone in a silent meditation with lapis lazuli, blue sodalite, or any other third eye chakra stone. Since Herkimer diamond can amplify thoughts and energy, make sure both stones have been cleansed beforehand. Hold Herkimer diamond in one hand and the remaining stone in the other as you allow divine wisdom to flow around and through you. This will create a vortex of powerful energy around your aura that will help stimulate your inner vision.

✦ INTUITIVE DREAM TOOL KIT ✦

FOR ENHANCING INTUITION

Moonstone

As its name suggests, moonstone shares a special connection to the moon and can be used in coordination with the lunar cycle. Due to the moon's association with emotions, the subconscious, and the divine feminine, moonstone carries a gentle and nurturing vibration that is perfect for harnessing your intuition post-dreams. Use it to tap into your inner feelings, raise your spiritual awareness, open the mind to new possibilities, and sense subtle shifts in your environment. Ultimately, moonstone wants you to know that your sensitivity is your superpower. Don't be afraid to use it.

Mini ritual: Though many variations of moonstone exist, we recommend using common moonstone for dreamwork. Use during a new moon for introspection or a full moon for illumination. Keep this stone handy by your bed and place it over your third eye chakra (located in the center of the forehead, between the brows) upon waking to facilitate a peaceful transition from sleep to consciousness. Perform this while lying in bed and remain silent for two to three minutes. Let any messages or images float up to the surface of your mind without judgment, then record your findings.

FOR UNCOVERING HIDDEN MESSAGES

Labradorite

Dreams work in mysterious ways, but so does labradorite. A favorite for dream recall, psychic development, and manifestation, labradorite is a gateway to your inner magic. With its dark gray base, labradorite may look like an ordinary stone, but upon tilting, a spectacular iridescent play of color appears, known as labradorescence, an effect that is named after this stone. These brilliant flashes of color will remind you that a simple shift in perspective can transform your life. This stone allows you to see the deeper meaning behind your experiences, reveals your hidden potential, and encourages you to embrace your shadows without fear.

Mini ritual: Use this stone to uncover the meaning behind confusing dream elements. With a particular dream symbol in mind, hold labradorite up to your third eye chakra to stimulate your inner vision. Allow your intuition to rise up and flow through this point in your body as you picture the symbol in your mind for one to two minutes. Pay attention to any feelings, words, or images that come up in response to the symbol, then examine them for deeper insight.

✦ INTUITIVE DREAM TOOL KIT ✦

FOR FILTERING OUT DISTRACTIONS

White Howlite

A stone of peace and spirituality, white howlite is a wonderful remedy for an overactive mind. Carrying a calming and patient energy, this stone is perfect for starting your morning with openness, clarity, and self-awareness. If you find that your brain is quick to jump to your to-do list for the day upon waking, use white howlite to quiet anxious or scattered thoughts and step into a place of active listening. By helping you slow down and find your center, this stone prepares you for receiving higher wisdom and intuitive messages during the interpretation process.

Mini ritual: Before interpreting your dreams, put any electronic devices away and find a quiet space to sit. Hold this stone in your hand and envision a white light softly shining down from above, starting at the top of your head. With each breath that you take, visualize the light traveling further down through your body until it is entirely filled with white light. In this space of stillness and receptivity, you can begin to interpret your dreams.

Affirmations

Daytime affirmations can support the interpretation process by promoting dream recall and activating your intuition. If you find your mind wandering to other thoughts at any point, use one of the following affirmations to gently ground your focus. Many of these affirmations can be used outside of dream interpretation too. Use them to create small moments of mindfulness throughout your day or whenever you need an intuitive boost.

AFFIRMATIONS

FOR DREAM RECALL

> My dream recall ability is growing stronger each day.

> The new insights I gain from my dreams are a catalyst for my personal growth and healing.

> When I recall my dreams with intention, my dream symbolism speaks to me loud and clear.

> My dreams are filled with powerful insights that I can access at anytime.

> When I approach my dreams with patience and gratitude, I unlock their deeper meaning and wisdom.

> I am free to explore and interpret my dreams at my own pace, in my own way.

> Remembering and interpreting my dreams feels natural and effortless.

FOR ELEVATING AWARENESS

> The answers I seek are unfolding beautifully before me, in alignment with divine timing.

> I am here. I am now. I am one with the present moment.

> I am open to new perspectives and revelations along my path of self-discovery.

> I shift my reality with conscious awareness and awakened presence.

> I am connected to my highest self, guardian angels, and spirit guides.

> I am discovering more about the true nature of my being every day.

> I am a vessel of infinite wisdom and universal knowledge.

FOR ACTIVATING INTUITION

> My intuition guides me in all ways, always.

> Whenever I feel uncertain, I remember the rich, internal reservoir of knowledge I have at my disposal and follow my instincts.

> I am discovering and embracing all the unique ways that my intuition speaks to me.

> In this moment, the best person to listen to is myself.

> My sensitivity is my superpower. The more I allow myself to feel, the stronger my intuition becomes.

> I release all doubt surrounding my intuitive abilities. I know myself. I trust myself.

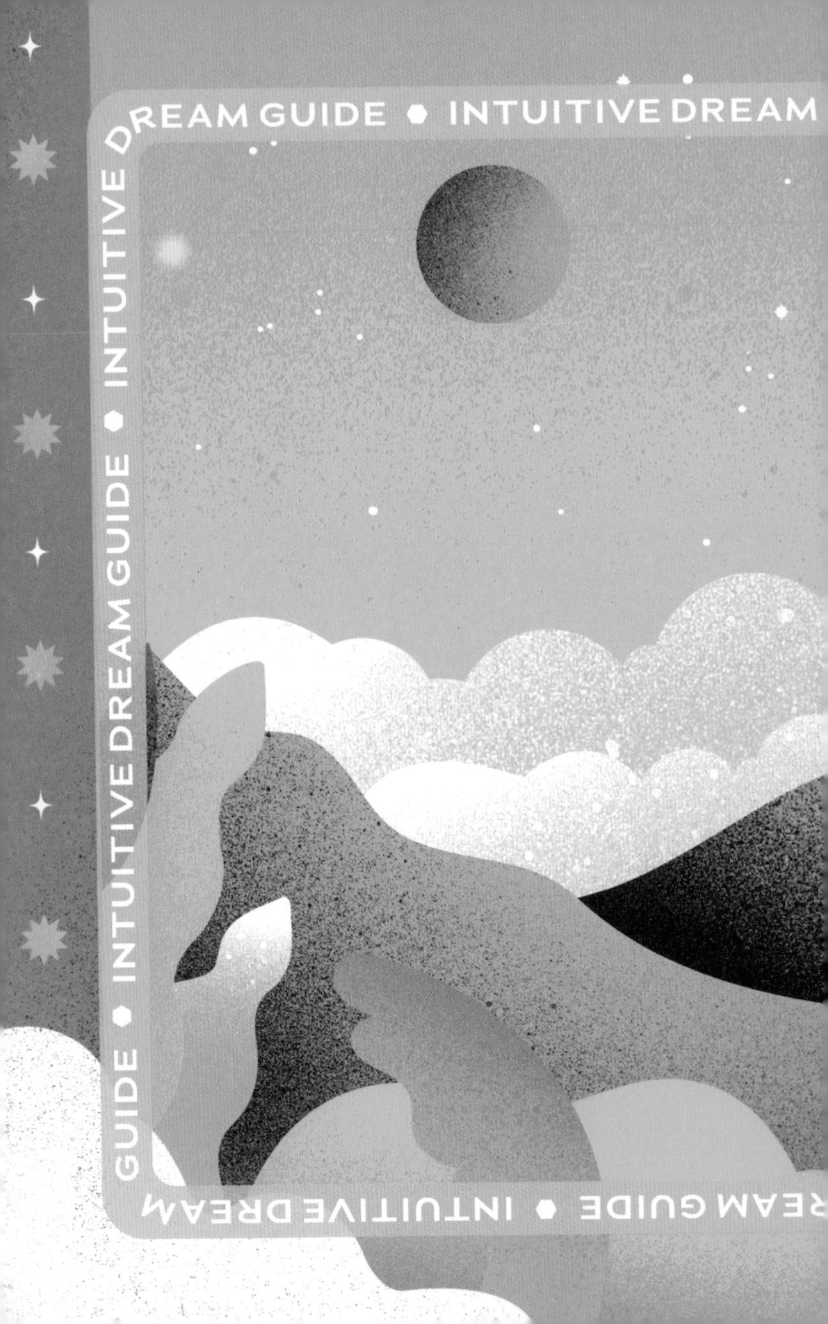

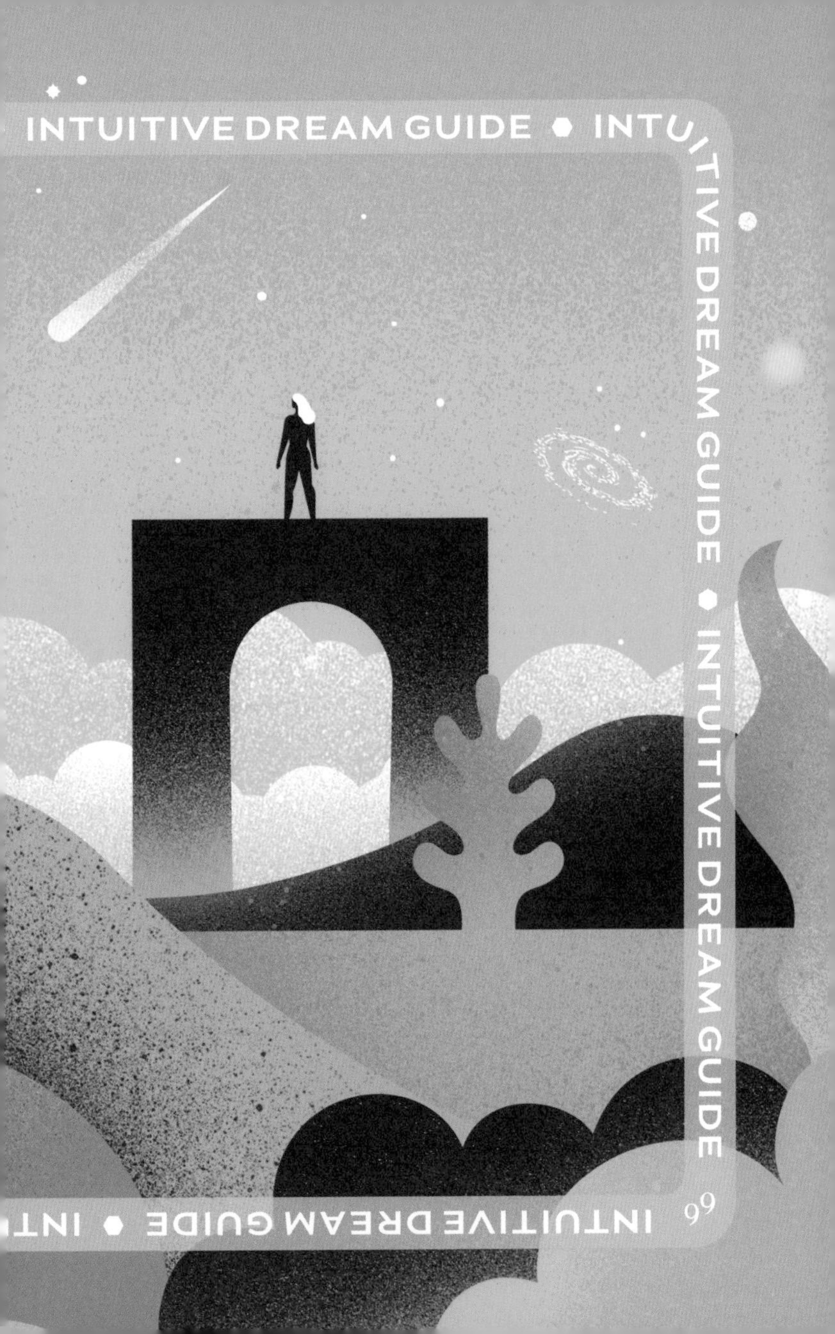
INTUITIVE DREAM GUIDE • INTUITIVE DREAM GUIDE • INTUITIVE DREAM GUIDE • INT

INTUITIVE DREAM GUIDE

Recording
Your Dreams

As vivid as your dreams may be, holding on to their details post-slumber can prove challenging. This is why promptly recording your dreams first thing in the morning is so important. Your dreams will be at their freshest and most memorable upon waking, and the more details you're able to immediately capture, the richer (and more illuminating) your interpretations will be. Here are a few tips and practices you can follow to ensure that nothing slips away.

———

SET ASIDE ALARM-FREE MORNINGS
TO RECORD DREAMS WHEN POSSIBLE

Though you can't always anticipate or plan for dreams, they are usually easier to remember when your body wakes up naturally and gradually. Because sudden alarms can disrupt your sleep cycle and easily displace dreams, it may be beneficial to set aside days when you can wake up without one.

KEEP A DREAM JOURNAL
NEXT TO YOUR BED

Having a pen and pad handy upon waking makes it easier
to jot down dreams. We recommend keeping a specially
designated dream journal by your bed so you can record
all of your dreams in one place. Doing so will not only
improve consistency but also help you spot recurring patterns and themes over time.

USE A TAPE RECORDER
AS AN ALTERNATIVE

If you struggle with writing in the morning or find that
your dream journal is out of reach, use a tape recorder
as a temporary alternative. Recording a voice memo on
your cell phone works too, just be sure to keep your eyes
closed once you've hit the record button so you don't get
distracted by the screen. Some may prefer this method to
writing, as it can help you remain still for longer and record
details faster.

WHEN YOU FIRST WAKE UP, KEEP YOUR
EYES CLOSED AND YOUR BODY STILL

Sunlight and movement can shift your attention away
from your dream, so continue to lie in bed quietly for a
couple of minutes. During this time, allow your dream to

stay on the surface of your mind, collecting any details that bubble up.

IMMEDIATELY AFTER, RECORD YOUR DREAM

Once you've summoned all the details that you can remember, immediately turn to your dream journal to record them. The longer you wait to write them down, the harder it'll be to recall them, so it's best to do so while they're still fresh in your mind.

WRITE IN THE PRESENT TENSE

Writing in the present tense can help you recall details from your dream by immediately "transporting" you back into the dream environment. By describing your dream as if it's happening again in real time, you'll be able to recount your experience much more clearly and vividly.

BE DESCRIPTIVE, BUT DON'T WORRY ABOUT FORMATTING

Use rich language to describe your dreams, but do so in a quick and efficient way. For some, this could look like small notes, bullet points, or writing shorthand. Your dreams do not need to be recorded in complete sentences or in sequential order—what's important is that you get all the essential information down. Remember, you can always go back and rewrite your dreams, fix spelling and grammar, or add details later.

FOCUS ON WRITING, NOT ANALYZING

As you record your dream, you may start to wonder what certain elements mean, but now is not the time for interpretation. Trying to extract the meaning of your dream prematurely can prevent you from recounting other important details, so only focus on recording what happened for now, rather than why.

JOT DOWN SIGNIFICANT DETAILS FIRST

What stands out the most in your dream? If a symbol or an image grabs your attention, be sure to write it down before it slips away. This includes, but is not limited to, specific words, messages, numbers, dates, times, and names of people or places. If something is particularly vivid or bizarre, it's usually important.

INCLUDE AS MANY
DETAILS AS YOU CAN

Even a tiny symbol can be meaningful, so write down everything you're able to remember, even if it doesn't seem significant. Pay attention to any people, places, and objects you encounter, as these are often key elements. If you can only remember a small snippet, that's OK!

WRITE DOWN ANY FEELINGS
OR SENSATIONS

Capturing the emotional content of your dream is vital to understanding its deeper meaning, so take note of any feelings or thoughts that occurred during the dream. Record shapes, textures, colors, or smells you come across too, as they can also inform your interpretation.

GIVE YOUR DREAM A TITLE

Oftentimes, the title of a dream can reveal a lot about its meaning, as how you choose to name it may point to an overarching theme or message. Naming your dream also makes it easier to remember. When naming your dream, don't overthink it—just use whatever comes to mind first. For example, if you had a dream about being stuck on a ship, you could title it "Lost at Sea" or "Rocky Waters."

DRAW YOUR DREAM (OPTIONAL)

If it's difficult for you to convey your dreams in writing, consider drawing them instead. Some people find it easier to express their dreams through images rather than words and may benefit from a visual approach. We recommend trying to capture your dreams through drawing and writing, as both are capable of delivering unique insights.

———

MEDITATE ON YOUR DREAM
LATER IN THE DAY

In the afternoon or evening, spend a few minutes in silent meditation to slow down and listen to your intuition. Taking this small break will provide space for any lingering dream insights to rise up, revealing details and perspectives you may have overlooked or not considered before.

———

BE CONSISTENT

With continued practice, you'll be able to recall your dreams more frequently. Record your dreams every day, or as often as you can. If you don't remember anything, simply write "No dreams today" in your journal. Combined with regular affirmations and the intention to remember your dreams, these daily recordings will support you in making dream journaling a natural habit.

Interpreting Your Dreams

Dreams are rich with personal meaning, making dream interpretation one of the most powerful tools of self-insight you have at your disposal. Although navigating the content of your dreams may feel strange at first, uncovering their secrets is simply a matter of following your intuition. By tapping into your senses, honoring your soul's truth, and embracing your inner wisdom, messages from your dreams can become a guiding force on your path of self-discovery.

Intuitive dream interpretation differs from other forms of dream analysis in that it focuses on amplifying and strengthening the intuitive voice. By peeling back layers of critical thought and opening a window to the subconscious, intuitive dream interpretation cultivates a connection to deeper states of awareness where you can explore your dreams, and their associations, more freely.

The following step-by-step guide will lead you through the nourishing process of intuitive dream interpretation, along with a series of gentle techniques designed to harness your intuition. Before you begin, understand that there is no need to translate your dream into a rational, linear message or "answer." Some of your dreams may point to a specific meaning, but others might not. If you can't seem to make sense of a particular dream, or dream symbol, it's OK to move on. Chances are, it may not have contained a message. Ultimately, your intuition will support you in sensing when something is worth investigation.

———

LET GO OF LIMITING BELIEFS

The first step to understanding your dreams is approaching them with an open mind. Dreams don't always make sense on the surface, but this doesn't mean you should dismiss them. Viewing your dreams as illogical or unimportant will only hold you back from discovering their true meaning, so adopt a nonjudgmental attitude from the start. Before reviewing your dream, be sure to release any negative thoughts, limiting beliefs, or reservations you may have about the process. Trust that your dreams will guide you, and they will.

———

INVOKE YOUR INTUITION AS A GUIDE

Once you're ready to explore the infinite potential of your dreams, take a moment to tap into your intuition. Find a quiet, distraction-free space where you can filter out the noise of the external world and drop into a place of deep, inner resonance. Be present with your feelings and make an effort to consciously carry them throughout the following steps. Understand that you are the ultimate authority on your dreams and that your intuition is your greatest ally. If you are experiencing intuitive roadblocks, refer back to our chapter on *How to Cultivate Your Intuition* (page 51).

––––

MAKE ASSOCIATIONS

After you've harnessed your intuition, review the most standout elements of your dream via free association, a technique designed to uncover subconscious and unconscious connections, thoughts, and feelings. Go over the main images, symbols, objects, characters, and settings of your dream piece by piece, allowing ideas, words, and memories to enter your mind freely. Write down everything that surfaces, then repeat the process for the other elements. When finished, reflect on the associations you've made and notice any connections. For example, if you dreamt of walking around your childhood mall, you might associate it with words such as *comfort, searching, home, growing pains, stagnation, young, restless,* and so on. From this, you may conclude that you are looking to move beyond your current comfort zone in the pursuit of riskier, yet more rewarding endeavors. If you get stuck on a particular symbol, visit our Dream Compass (page 149) for additional perspectives to inspire your interpretations.

———

IDENTIFY EMOTIONS

Now that you're aware of what certain dream elements may represent, consider the emotional tone of the dream. Were you excited? Afraid? Anxious? Was there a disconnect between how you think you should have felt and what you actually did feel? Did you notice any smells, sounds, colors, shapes, or sensations? If anything evoked an emotional response in the dream, ask yourself why. Identifying these emotions and examining their root cause can lead you to a more meaningful interpretation. For instance, if you had a dream about being chased through the woods and the primary emotion was fear, what exactly in the dream made you fearful? Was it the specific pursuer, the consequences of getting caught, or having to navigate unfamiliar terrain in the dark? Honing in on these connections can provide further insights.

———

MAKE COMPARISONS TO WAKING LIFE

To uncover the larger meaning of your dream, think about the type of reality or "truth" that is being revealed to you.

Because many dreams are based upon what you experience during the day, examining its themes in relation to current life events can provide greater context. For example, consider a dream about climbing up multiple, wobbly flights of stairs. Although the stairs were unstable, you were still able to ascend them successfully. This dream illustrates a reality where upward mobility and progress are possible with concentrated effort, despite challenges in the environment. In the context of waking life, this may speak to rising above an obstacle at work or overcoming a "shaky" sense of confidence.

PAUSE AND ASK QUESTIONS

During this stage of the interpretation process, or at any other point, give yourself space to pause and ask questions. Answers won't always be obvious, so remove any pressure from yourself to gain immediate clarity. If you start to get frustrated or feel like you've hit a dead end, simply move on to another part of your dream or try asking a different question. The interpretation process is all about getting into a gentle, intuitive flow, so if you feel like you're forcing an answer, take a minute to step back and redirect your focus.

HONOR THE DREAM
THROUGH A RITUAL

Honoring your dream through a physical ritual is a great way to integrate subconscious lessons into your conscious, waking life. Performing a small physical act, such as saying an affirmation aloud, lighting a candle, or writing a note of gratitude for your dream, can help anchor its energy in the material realm beyond just merely thinking about it.

———

REVIEW YOUR DREAMS REGULARLY

The more you review your dreams, the more they'll reveal. Looking back through your dreams periodically makes it easier to recognize recurring themes and patterns that are playing out in your life. Not only that, but new details and perspectives may become more apparent to you during a second read-through, which could give your dream a different meaning. You may find that a message suddenly "clicks" or you can clearly see a situation for what it is.

Dream Elements

Although they don't always follow a narrative in the conventional, linear sense, dreams are like stories in that they use similar elements to convey a message or lesson. When interpreting a dream, it can be helpful to break down its individual components, such as its settings, characters, symbols, and emotional content, to distill important clues. Here's how you can begin to approach each element and understand its meaning.

SETTINGS

Every dream begins with a setting. Without a time and place, no story can exist. Settings indicate when and where a story occurs, and like all dream elements, they are symbolic. Many believe that a dream's location reflects one's inner psychological landscape, providing a visual portrayal of their current mindset or state of being. For instance, dreaming of a barren desert could represent feelings of isolation or detachment, while a stormy sea could illustrate turbulent emotions. Dream settings can also speak to an aspect of life you are subconsciously processing.

To determine its meaning, examine both the "time element" and the "place element" of your dream. What do you associate with the period of life you're being shown? What personal connections do you have to the location? Consider your history with the setting, if applicable, as well as the architecture of the dream. Dream architecture refers to how a dream environment is structured. Large spaces may represent big-picture aspects of life, while small spaces may point to everyday matters. Likewise, a clean, open atmosphere may signal clear thinking or mental freedom, while a cramped and cluttered environment may depict disorganized or overwhelming thoughts.

CHARACTERS

Characters in a dream are like actors in a play, each with a different role. They speak to the dynamics of your life and add multiple perspectives to the dream. Characters can represent subjects and ideas, embody archetypes, and personify your inner thoughts, feelings, and perceptions. Essentially, they are walking, talking symbols. More often than not, the people you see or become in your dream represent an aspect of yourself, so keep this in mind during interpretation. And remember, looks can be deceiving! A character's outward appearance is typically a "mask" for something deeper, so while your dreams may depict people you know, understand that it's not really "them." Familiar figures within dreams are usually a manifestation of some part of yourself, so consider the qualities they reflect in you, as well as the nature of your relationship, rather than your personal connection to them. For instance, your maternal self might manifest as your mother or a very nurturing friend, while your professional self might appear as a boss, a coworker, or an employee.

Besides exploring these links, you can also think of characters as an emotional, physical, mental, or spiritual expression of yourself. For example, a teacher or student may represent an intellectual or mental aspect of yourself and embody your desire for knowledge, while a doctor could be seen as your healing self and speak to your spiritual nature. For additional clues, observe your interactions with the character(s), and how you respond to them emotionally. If you dreamt of protecting a baby, for example, this could be interpreted as you shielding a vulnerable side of yourself, safeguarding a newborn business, or holding on to your own innocence.

SYMBOLS

A picture is worth a thousand words, and the same can be said about dream symbols. After all, symbolism is the language of dreams. A symbol is anything that stands for, or represents, something else, such as an object, a word, a number, a color, a character, or a setting. Typically, symbols are used to express something abstract, like a concept or an idea (e.g., harmony, fear, a desire for adventure, etc.). While some symbols are universal, the meaning of a symbol is ultimately personal. Symbols mean different things to different people, depending on their personal experiences and point of view, so the only way to interpret them is to determine what rings true for you.

When approaching this element of dreams, it's important to examine both the symbol itself and the action and context of the "scene." Consider the symbol of water, for example. On its own, water can represent many things—emotions, cleansing, change, healing, and more. But what does it say about your dream? Without knowing the action and context involved, it's impossible to tell.

Luckily, as the dreamer, all of this information is right before your eyes. You just have to learn how to "read" it. For instance, watering a garden in a dream may illustrate the process of nourishing your emotional foundation, while swimming upstream could be seen as fighting against your emotions. In both dreams, water is symbolic of emotions, yet the symbolism of the scenes gives each an entirely different meaning. Additionally, symbols can hold multiple meanings simultaneously, so don't be afraid to explore different angles. For example, swimming upstream may not only be a metaphor for resisting your feelings but may also represent a situation that feels like an uphill battle. Whenever you encounter a new symbol, record it and what it means to you personally in the back of your dream journal to create your very own dream dictionary or glossary. Use it as a reference for future dreams if you come across repeating symbols.

EMOTIONS

When intuitively interpreting your dreams, your emotions reign supreme. This is because emotions are a massive indicator of what a dream symbol represents. Think about it: Every piece of your dream—whether the settings, characters, or symbols—serves as a type of "mask." As projections of your inner world, they almost always require you to dig beneath their surface, and thus, can rarely be taken at face value. However, quite the opposite is true of emotions. Emotions in dreams are usually never disguised. They aren't a metaphor that needs translating or a facade for something else. The feelings in your dreams reflect your *true, honest* feelings (including those that are subconscious or repressed), which makes them a reliable source of guidance.

That said, examining your emotional responses to different elements of your dream can open up a new perspective and shed light on their true meaning. For example, seeing a cat in a dream isn't inherently "good" or "bad." Although its appearance (clean, scraggly, young, etc.) can inform you of certain qualities, it's how you *feel* about the cat that matters. Does the cat make you feel scared, frustrated, or curious? Identify the emotions involved, and then ask yourself why. Oftentimes, these feelings mirror your emotions in waking life. For instance, being afraid of a dying cat in a dream may point to fears of your own mortality, while feeling relief may indicate that you're ready to release an old part of yourself or move past an unhealthy situation.

Dream Template

Ready to put what you've learned into action? Use the following Dream Template to get started. This template will walk you through the basic steps of recording and interpreting a dream. It consists of two parts: "My Dream" (for recording details) and "My Interpretation" (for interpreting its meaning). As you work through the prompts, record your answers in a separate dream journal or on a blank piece of paper; do not write directly in the book, as there's only one template provided here. Keep in mind that some parts of the template may not be applicable to your specific dream, so feel free to skip over anything that doesn't resonate. To better understand how this process works, follow along with the filled-in Dream Template Example at the end of the section for additional guidance. As always, we encourage you to follow your intuition and make this template your own, so modify or expand upon it however you see fit.

MY DREAM

DATE:

DREAM TITLE:

WHAT STANDS OUT THE MOST:

The most memorable, vivid, or strangest part of your dream. This may include but is not limited to numbers, dates and times, names of people and places, specific words, messages or instructions, symbols, images, and objects.

DREAM SYMBOLS AND IMAGES:

Anything that appears within your dream. Record the most significant ones first and include as much detail as possible.

WHERE AND WHEN IT IS:

The setting of your dream. Describe the location (e.g., childhood home, futuristic hospital, brother's tenth birthday party, etc.), time period, and atmosphere.

WHO IS PRESENT:

The characters in your dream. These could be people, animals, or other figures.

WHAT IS HAPPENING:

The action or "plot" of your dream. Note: Your dream may not have a plot. Resist the urge to create one if none exists, as the conscious mind may try to fabricate a narrative.

HOW I FEEL (IN THE DREAM):

The emotions and sensations you experience in your dream. Record any feelings, thoughts, sounds, smells, tastes, colors, or textures.

HOW I FEEL NOW:

The emotions and sensations you are currently experiencing.

HOW I FELT BEFORE BED:

The emotions and sensations you experienced before going to sleep.

KEYWORDS/THEME:

Choose three words to describe your dream or its core theme.

RECURRING DREAM:

■ yes
■ no

SLEEP QUALITY:

●·············●·············●
1   5   10

DRAW IT:

MY INTERPRETATION

WHAT DO I ASSOCIATE WITH EACH
DREAM SYMBOL OR IMAGE?

*Focus on one symbol or image at a time, writing down any words,
thoughts, and memories that come to mind. Repeat this for as many
dream elements as desired.*

WHAT DOES THE SETTING OF
MY DREAM MEAN TO ME?

*Draw connections between the dream setting and areas of your life,
moments in time, and your own psychological landscape.*

WHAT IS MY RELATIONSHIP TO
THE CHARACTERS IN MY DREAM?

Examine your interactions and feelings toward any characters and consider what they may represent. They are usually projections of your inner world.

WHAT DOES THE EMOTIONAL TONE
OF MY DREAM INDICATE?

Observe your emotional responses to various dream elements to uncover what they symbolize. Pay attention to how you felt before and how you feel after the dream for additional clues.

WHAT COMPARISONS CAN
I DRAW FROM WAKING LIFE?

Consider whether current events in your life may be influencing your dream. Recurring themes and patterns in your dream could point to a real-life situation or issue that needs to be addressed.

FINAL THOUGHTS:

Record any conclusions or what you believe the dream is trying to tell you.

Dream Template Example

MY DREAM

DATE:

8/4

DREAM TITLE:

Breaking Free

WHAT STANDS OUT THE MOST:

Bird breaking out from the skin under my knee

DREAM SYMBOLS AND IMAGES:

Yellow bird's beak, knee

WHERE AND WHEN IT IS:

Doctor's office, present day

WHO IS PRESENT:

A doctor and my boyfriend

WHAT IS HAPPENING:

I am sitting at the doctor's office and some type of bird (chicken, eagle, or vulture?) is underneath my flesh. It's trying to peck its way out through my kneecap. It has a very pronounced, sharp yellow beak. I put my knee up and am waiting for the doctor to remove it but my boyfriend is also there, helping me. Eventually, my boyfriend takes it out but when he does, another bird is right behind it.

HOW I FEEL (IN THE DREAM):

Confused, anxious

HOW I FEEL NOW:

Relieved

HOW I FELT BEFORE BED:

A little tired

KEYWORDS/THEME:

Liberation, freedom, breaking barriers

RECURRING DREAM:

☐ yes

☒ no

SLEEP QUALITY:

1   5   10

DRAW IT:

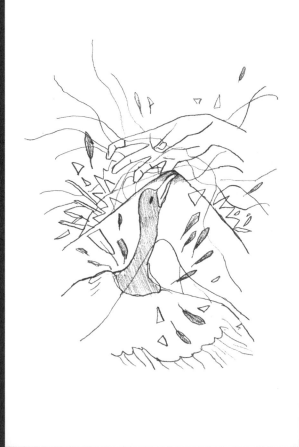

MY INTERPRETATION

WHAT DO I ASSOCIATE WITH EACH DREAM SYMBOL OR IMAGE?

Bird - freedom, soaring, rising above, leaving the nest

Beak - resourcefulness, self-expression, ability to take in nourishment

Knee - stability, movement, vulnerability, surrender

WHAT DOES THE SETTING OF MY DREAM MEAN TO ME?

Could be related to health or healing. Shows that I am subconsciously seeking help or answers regarding a problem. The mood is tense. There's a sense of urgency and need to "fix" the situation.

WHAT IS MY RELATIONSHIP TO THE CHARACTERS IN MY DREAM?

I view the doctor and my boyfriend as healing forces because the doctor is a healing professional and my boyfriend is a nurse in real life. Both are trying to assist me in removing the bird. They could represent my "inner healer" or spiritual guidance/assistance that I have at my disposal. The bird may symbolize a part of myself that wishes to be liberated, or a new idea or way of thinking that is beginning to surface.

WHAT DOES THE EMOTIONAL TONE OF MY DREAM INDICATE?

There is uncertainty surrounding how to let a new aspect of myself emerge. I am anxious to move forward (shown by the doctor and my boyfriend rushing to help me), yet fearful about how to navigate the process (I don't feel confident removing the bird myself). The situation makes me feel uncomfortable, but I know I need to do something about it. The bird can't stay under my skin, and it obviously doesn't want to. Maybe a feeling I've been ignoring is starting to bubble over?

WHAT COMPARISONS CAN I DRAW TO WAKING LIFE?

Recently, I've been thinking about quitting my job to pursue photography full time. I like the security my current job offers, but I'm starting to feel stifled. I think I'm beginning to realize how much I value having creative freedom over my work, but I'm scared to make the jump and switch careers. This dream seems to relate to breaking out of my comfort zone and allowing my true needs to come to light.

FINAL THOUGHTS:

I feel like this dream is about my subconscious desire for liberation. It shows that I have the tools I need to free myself (the bird's beak), which I can use to move past my insecurities (the knee, which is a vulnerable/weak point on the body) and emerge as my most authentic self (the free bird). I think that another bird appears behind the first one that is removed because freeing myself is an ongoing process, not a onetime event. Doubts and fears will always creep in, but if I embrace my abilities, I can push through any limiting beliefs I've constructed in my mind. I think this dream is ultimately telling me to stop doubting myself and to pursue a career that will actually make me happy.

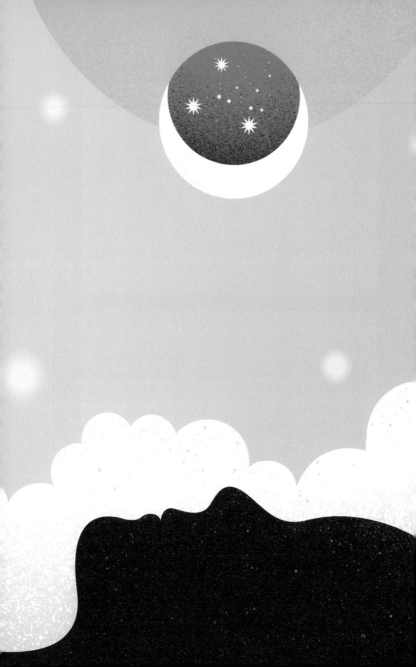

Journal Prompts

Navigating the content of your dreams is a process of self-inquiry, and questions are a great place to start. Asking questions allows you to extract vital information about different elements of your dream by helping you dig beneath their surface meaning. If you get stuck at any point or are unsure of what to ask, use the following journal prompts to uncover new details and perspectives. Some of these questions may or may not apply to your dream, so feel free to expand beyond them if you desire, and remember to follow your gut! If you find yourself pulled toward a specific question or thought, lean in and explore.

FOR DREAM SETTINGS

> What does the "time" of the setting mean to me? What do I associate with this period of my life?

> What does the "place" of the setting mean to me? Does the location have any personal significance?

> How would I describe the setting? Does its atmosphere or "mood" reflect my current mindset or state of being?

> How does the setting make me feel? If it's a familiar place, what emotions do I associate with it (e.g., comfort, fear, stress)?

> Does the setting have a specific function (e.g., a school is a place of learning)? What areas of life or subjects does it speak to?

> How am I viewing the setting (from above, below, far away, or close)? What does my perspective suggest?

> Have I dreamt of this place before? If so, when did it occur and what were the potential triggers?

FOR DREAM CHARACTERS

> What stands out about the character the most? Do any of their features seem exaggerated or out of place? If so, are these qualities I lack or desire in myself?

> What are the physical attributes of the character? Notice their age, clothing, stature, etc. What does their outer appearance suggest?

> How much independence, personality, and intelligence do they have? The more they have, the more important they may be to the dream.

> What actions does the character take, and how do I respond? Would I react the same way in real life or differently?

> How does the character make me feel?

> What does the character symbolize to me? What part of myself could they represent?

> Is the character a manifestation of a physical, mental, emotional, or spiritual aspect of myself?

> Does the character embody an archetype or stand for an abstract concept (e.g., my inner child, death, a force of nature, etc.)?

> Do I know the character in real life? If so, what is the nature of our relationship? What qualities or aspects of myself do they reflect?

FOR DREAM SYMBOLS

> Which symbols are the most significant? What is memorable about them?

> What does the symbol mean to me personally?

> What words do I associate with the symbol?

> What is the context of the symbol? How does it appear in my dream? What is it doing, and how and where is it doing it?

> Can the symbol be used it real life? What is its function? Does it work as it's supposed to?

> How do I feel about the symbol? What is my emotional response to it?

> When was the last time I encountered this symbol in real life, if at all?

> What comparisons can be drawn between my dream's symbolism and waking life?

FOR DREAM EMOTIONS

> What emotions did I experience in the dream? What caused them?

> Did I notice any shapes, colors, sounds, smells, textures, or tastes in my dream? How do they make me feel?

> When have I recently felt these emotions in my waking life? Is there a connection between my dream scenario and a real-world situation?

> How do I usually deal with these emotions? Do I make space to honor and process them or tend to ignore them?

> What do these emotions feel like in my body? What physical sensations do they evoke and where?

> How did I feel before going to sleep? Does my emotional state before bed correlate with my post-dream feelings?

Once you've assessed the individual elements of your dream, don't forget to combine the pieces! Consider how the setting relates to the characters and symbols, and what each part contributes to the message as a whole. This will give you a deeper understanding of what your dream means.

Intuitive Rituals

Rituals are actions we imbue with meaning and intention. When performed with awareness, energy, and presence, they transform the mundane into the sacred. Even a simple act, such as drinking a cup of tea, can be a power- ful ritual if done with purpose. While rituals don't have to be long or complex, carving out time for them can greatly enhance your dream interpretation practice and support mindfulness in general. Use them to slow down, clear your mind, and reflect. Here are three intuitive rituals that every dreamer needs in their tool kit.

THIRD EYE CHAKRA
ACTIVATION RITUAL

Materials: a piece of amethyst (or your favorite purple crystal), pen, and notepad

The third eye chakra, also known as the brow chakra, is considered the seat of your intuitive wisdom. It is associated with foresight, openness, imagination, and higher realms of consciousness. It also shares a link to the pineal gland, which helps regulate biorhythms, such as sleep and wake times. If you're having difficulty seeing the bigger picture behind your dreams, use the following ritual to open and activate your intuition.

1. Lie down on a bed or a comfortable surface and place your crystal on your third eye chakra (in the center of the forehead, between the brows). Close your eyes.

2. Take ten deep breaths, releasing any tension or tightness in your body with every exhale. Repeat this until you feel completely at ease.

3. With your eyes still closed, focus on the feeling of the crystal against your skin. Imagine it softly humming with energy connecting you to your inner wisdom. Then envision a small, white ball of light glowing above your third eye.

4. Visualize the ball slowly growing larger and brighter as your connection to your intuition grows stronger. Watch it change from a soft white shade to a majestic, deep purple color.

5. When you feel like you've fully harnessed your intuition, ask yourself, "What does my intuition want me to see in this moment?" Then remove the crystal and open your eyes. Journal your thoughts afterward. Keep the crystal somewhere visible to remind you that your intuition will always guide you.

FULL MOON ILLUMINATION AND RELEASE RITUAL

Materials: a piece of moonstone, bay leaf
or small piece of paper, pen, candle, bowl,
and nonflammable dish

Full moons are an especially potent time for dreamwork, as they represent the energetic peak of the monthly lunar cycle. The light of this phase serves to amplify and heighten your vision and emotions, allowing for break-throughs in perspective and greater clarity. Perform this ritual during the full moon to release limiting beliefs, reveal the truth behind illusions, and attract insightful dreams. To determine the date of the next full moon, consult a lunar calendar online.

1. Find a quiet place to sit and meditate with your crystal in your dominant hand for five minutes. Slow your breathing and focus on harnessing your intuition.

2. When you feel connected, ask yourself, "What must I release in order to embrace my truth?" This could be fear, doubt, anxiety, limiting beliefs, negativity, or toxic habits.

3. Set your crystal aside, then write down on a bay leaf an intention to release whatever is no longer serving you, such as "I release self-doubt." A small piece of paper can be used as an alternative.

4. Place your candle in a bowl or shallow dish with water for safety. Light the candle. Focus on the flame and its purifying essence. With your intention clear in your mind, touch the bay leaf to the flame while saying your intention aloud. Once lit, transfer the leaf to a nonflammable dish and let it fully burn. Continue to repeat your intention until the flame goes out.

5. Allow the candle to burn down on its own or snuff it out before bed with a candle snuffer. If using a jar candle, place a lid on the jar to smother the flame. Light the candle on subsequent days until it burns down completely to continue calling in guidance from your dreams.

SOOTHING WATERS RITUAL BATH

Materials: carrier oil, lavender essential oil, Epsom salts, fresh or dried rose petals, candles, a piece of amethyst, and a cup of tea (optional)

Water has been used as an energetic cleanser throughout history due to its purifying, renewing, and healing properties. It also acts as a conduit for Spirit by enhancing your connection to the universe. Taking a ritual bath is a beautiful act of cleansing that allows you to bathe with a spiritual purpose or intention. Use it to wash away the stress of the day and create an oasis of calm within your life. Set aside twenty to sixty minutes of uninterrupted time for this ritual.

1. Draw a bath. Mix one teaspoon of your favorite carrier oil with five drops of lavender essential oil. Add it to the water with one heaping scoop of Epsom salts, a handful of rose petals, and any other herbs or flowers you desire.

2. Turn down the lights and light some candles. Before getting into the tub, meditate with the amethyst in your hands and close your eyes. Connect with its calming energy and breathe deeply and slowly for one minute.

3. When ready, say aloud, "I nourish the tides of my emotions. I allow myself to feel, heal, and be held by love." Then step into the tub. Submerge yourself completely beneath the water, letting it cleanse you of negativity, attachments, judgments, and expectations.

4. As you surface, imagine you are rebirthing yourself, feeling pure and refreshed as you emerge from the water. Continue bathing and visualize the rose petals as glowing pink hearts, surrounding and filling you with a vibration of unconditional love.

5. When finished, get out of the tub and watch the water flow down the drain, carrying away all that no longer serves you. Allow yourself to drip-dry to prolong the energetic effects of the bath.

6. Place the amethyst under your pillow to create a calming sleep environment and encourage peaceful dreams. If desired, enjoy a cup of tea before bed, such as chamomile or passion-flower tea, to support further relaxation.

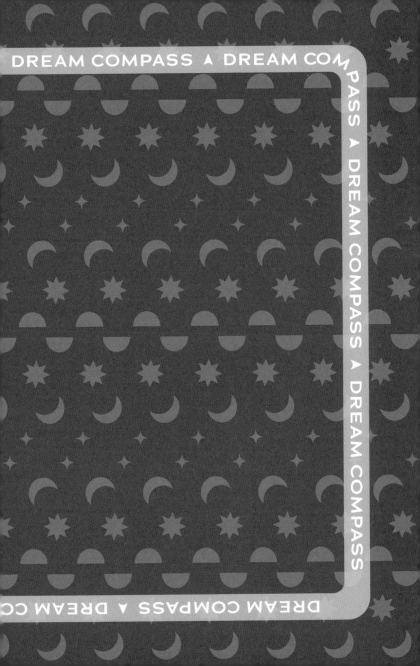

DREAM COMPASS

A Guide to Common Dream Symbols and Scenarios

If you need some help interpreting the symbols that show up in your dreams, our Dream Compass is here to guide your intuition home. Unlike a dream dictionary (which often includes specific and narrow definitions for symbols), the Dream Compass is designed to encourage an expansive, open-ended approach to interpreting the most common dream symbols and scenarios. Each symbol opens with a brief overview of common interpretations for the symbol, followed by open-ended prompts to help you use your intuition and enrich your own lines of questioning for deep, personal insight.

Keep in mind, there is no single definitive meaning for any dream symbol. No symbol is inherently "good" or "bad." It all boils down to how you personally relate to it. So while our Dream Compass can be used to understand major themes and associations, think of the following as soft guidelines rather than hard rules. They can point out different paths, but it's up to you to choose. Always look to the emotional content of your dream for clues to a symbol's meaning.

ANT

The ant is a symbol of hard work, determination, patience, teamwork, and unity. Despite its tiny size, some species can lift up to five thousand times their own body weight, demonstrating their immense strength. Positive interactions with ants in a dream may indicate that you are persevering toward your goals, while negative interactions may point to petty annoyances in life that have grown into larger problems.

———

Ants are a reminder that things take time to come to fruition. Instead of focusing on reaching an end goal, be aware of your current thoughts and actions, as they ultimately influence how you get to your destination. Patience is key.

———

The saying "it takes a village" implies that many people must cooperate to achieve a common goal. Look to themes involving community and collaboration for greater clues. The number of ants can also shed light on feelings of isolation (single ant) or a desire to belong (many ants).

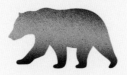

BEAR

The bear is a symbol of strength, courage, confidence, and grounding forces. Seeing this animal in a dream may signal that it's time to stand up for yourself. On the other hand, the bear can also represent a call for rest, solitude, or introspection, due to its strong connection to the earth element.

———

How do you overcome adversity? Leading from a place of courage and strength can inspire the same in others. The challenges you're currently facing may even be preparing you for a position of leadership. Lean into their lessons.

———

Bears are typically solitary animals, emphasizing themes of privacy and boundaries. Many of them also hibernate during the winter months, highlighting a need for rest. If you've been busy, this may be a sign to slow down. Schedule some alone time to connect to your higher self. A silent meditation in nature can allow messages to be heard.

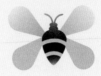

BEE

An industrious species, bees are considered the world's most important pollinator and are an integral part of most ecosystems. Generally seen as a favorable sign, bees are thought to symbolize good fortune, happiness, hard work, harmony, order, and abundance. If you've been diligently working toward your goals, there's a good chance your efforts are about to pay off. If not, your mounting responsibilities could be causing some anxiety. Look to issues surrounding work-life balance or social dynamics for further clues.

Does your current workload challenge you in exciting ways, or is it beginning to feel like a burden? Do your daily accomplishments bring you a sense of pride? Consider what you've been building toward and whether it still fulfills you on a soul level.

Bees live in a highly organized society. Seeing bees could indicate that it's time to fine-tune the existing structures in your life and get your responsibilities in order. Since bees are social creatures, reviewing the health of your friendships, group associations, and joint collaborations could also prove fruitful.

BIRD

Birds primarily symbolize freedom due to their ability to traverse the Earth and skies. Other common themes include perspective, vision, agility, movement, and individuality. Different species of birds carry various meanings, so researching the type you encounter will provide more context. For instance, the dove is a symbol of hope.

Seeing a bird may indicate transitions in your life. Are you ready to spread your wings and fly? Think of where you may be able to apply more flexibility and adaptability in order to reach new heights.

Birds are associated with the element of air, which represents communication, intellect, and knowledge. Are you being intentional with your thoughts and words? Speaking reflectively and thinking things through may help get a situation or an idea off the ground if you've been stuck.

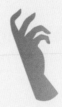

BODY PARTS

Body parts generally deal with an aspect of one's ego, conscious identity, or health. Those that appear different in a dream are particularly significant. To unpack their meaning, examine the function of each part and what it contributes to the body as a whole. Tuning into any physical sensations around these areas may also help pinpoint hidden issues or feelings.

———

Shoulders or the spine may correlate with responsibility, breasts with nourishment, bones with one's ancestral roots, ankles with support and direction, feet with mobility and independence, eyes with vision, and ears with receptivity.

———

Dead or severed body parts can be frightening to encounter in a dream, but their removal or destruction may be a sign that change is needed. Think about what you can eliminate from your life to make new room for growth.

BOOK

Books represent information, knowledge, truth, and wisdom. Seeing a book in a dream could mean that you are seeking knowledge in your waking life or that you have a desire to learn something new.

———

Consider the appearance of the book and what it says about your current mindset. An open book may indicate a willingness to accept new ideas, while a closed book could signify hidden depths. Reading an old book could imply that memories from the past are on your mind.

———

Examine your interactions with the book for greater context. Are you writing a new chapter, searching for answers, or using it to escape from reality? What role do you play in your own story? Think about the narrative you've written for yourself and whether it accurately reflects who you are.

BUTTERFLY OR MOTH

At its core, the butterfly (or moth) is emblematic of change, signaling personal transformation. Developing through a process called metamorphosis, it goes from egg to caterpillar to chrysalis or cocoon, and finally, to adult. Seeing a butterfly in a dream may be asking you to look to the seasons, cycles, and rhythms of your own life. Are you aware of your evolution? Do you appreciate the beauty that is unfolding each day, within and around you?

———

The butterfly speaks to a lightness of being or playfulness. If your spirit feels heavy or burdened, this could be a sign to cultivate more joy and fun in your life. It may also indicate a need to look at conflicting situations from a more lighthearted perspective.

———

Noticing where in the life cycle your butterfly is can provide clues to its meaning. Did it start out as a butterfly, caterpillar, or cocoon in your dream? Draw parallels to waking life and how you can step into the next phase of being that you desire.

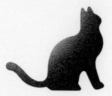

CAT

Throughout history, cats have been strongly associated with magic, mystery, and the unconscious. Some cultures regard cats as symbols of good fortune, while others perceive them to be a sign of evil or deceit. The ancient Egyptians deeply revered cats and worshipped numerous cat-like goddesses, supporting a connection between cats and women. With such wide-ranging connotations, cats remain somewhat of a secretive symbol, but they likely point to a hidden nature or an area of untapped potential.

———

Consider the major feminine figures or influences that are currently in your life, as well as your connection to your own feminine energy. Are there hidden intentions you may not be aware of? Are you afraid of embracing your personal power or innate talents?

———

Observe your relationship to your intuition and primal instincts. Do you tend to trust them or ignore them? In dangerous situations, cats often seem to land on their feet, resulting in phrases such as "a cat has nine lives" and "cat-like reflexes." Following your gut may be the key to avoiding future pitfalls. Be confident in your next steps.

CHASE

Dreams of being chased may indicate that you are avoiding something in your waking life. Instead of confronting an issue head-on, you've chosen to flee, but more often than not, this only delays the inevitable. If you've been in denial about a situation or shirking your responsibilities, such dreams may be a sign that a problem is getting worse. Be mindful of any escapist tendencies you may subconsciously be indulging in.

———

Notice who or what is pursuing you and what they may represent. This could be an aspect of yourself you are choosing to ignore, feelings that you have rejected, changes you refuse to accept, or anything you perceive to be a threat. This can even include love if you fear being vulnerable.

———

Consider the distance between you and your pursuer, as your proximity to one another may mirror how close you are to a problem. Widening the gap between you and the other could imply that you are distancing yourself from the issue or that it is finally resolving. However, if the pursuer is catching up to you, this may signify that the situation is impending and will not go away until you choose to deal with it.

CHEATING ON A PARTNER

Dreaming of cheating on a partner can be interpreted a number of ways. While such dreams tend to highlight relationship issues, they are rarely about actual cheating and may not have anything to do with your love life. Cheating dreams may represent any situation where you felt dishonest, guilty, or unfulfilled to a certain extent.

Have you compromised your integrity, beliefs, or ideals recently? Your dream may be encouraging you to review any instances of self-betrayal. If you are prone to self-sabotage, it could be a sign of more deeply rooted fears surrounding trust, self-esteem, or abandonment.

Are you being truthful with your current needs? If an aspect of your relationship isn't satisfying you, repressed desires could manifest as this type of dream. Opening up a dialogue with your significant other and discussing how to better fulfill your needs can allow your relationship to grow.

CLOCK

Generally, a clock symbolizes the passage of time. It speaks to mortality, transitions, beginnings, endings, and finite resources. Seeing a clock in a dream may be reminding you to spend your time and energy wisely. It also could be highlighting projects or situations that are causing a feeling of time pressure.

———

Have you been procrastinating? A clock could represent a looming deadline or task that's been causing anxiety or a feeling of unpreparedness. Consider the first steps you can take to address the issue.

———

What do you value in life? Your career, health, or time with friends and family? Think about where your priorities lie and whether you're carving out ample time for them. Reassessing your pace and commitments and ensuring they're sustainable will serve you well in the long run.

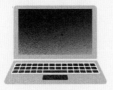

COMPUTER

Computers symbolize technology and information. Like the human brain, they retrieve, store, and transmit data. In this sense, a computer may represent how you think. Seeing a functional computer in a dream could speak to your ability to access information, while a broken computer might point to an overworked mind, limiting thoughts, or conflicting internal opinions.

———

Dreaming about technology can point to a desire to make life more efficient. Think about ways you can better handle issues or shave time off your current tasks. Your methods of problem solving may also be up for review.

———

Are you being receptive to all sources of knowledge? This could be a sign that you need to expand your mind and seek information elsewhere, especially if you've felt mentally blocked lately.

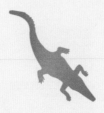

CROCODILE OR ALLIGATOR

Stealthy, efficient, and ferocious, crocodiles and alligators have roamed the Earth for over eighty million years, making them a symbol of ancient wisdom. As apex predators, they represent sovereignty and independence. Crocodiles are successful because they know when to wait and when to strike. Patience and perseverance are key.

———

Are you biting off more than you can chew? If your interaction with the crocodile was negative, you may want to reconsider your plan of attack regarding a current situation. Don't pick battles that will completely exhaust your efforts or affect your performance. Be patient and wait for an opportune moment.

———

Both the crocodile and the alligator work with water energy, which symbolizes emotions. Are you being true to your authentic feelings? An inner well of wisdom is at your disposal if you're willing to look beyond the surface.

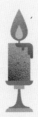

DEATH

Dreams about death or dying usually speak to profound internal changes, as well as themes of self-discovery, transformation, and personal growth. With every ending comes a new beginning, so this dream may be a sign that you're moving on from old habits or ways of thinking and stepping into a new chapter of life or a different mindset.

———

If someone you know dies in your dream, it could indicate that an aspect of your relationship is changing, but more often than not, this person tends to represent a part of yourself. Consider the qualities they reflect in you and whether these pieces have changed.

———

If you're the person who dies in your dream, you may be going through a major transitional period in your life. Endings pave the way for new growth, so think about what needs to be released in order for you to move forward. Death can also be seen as a wake-up call if you've been avoiding or attempting to escape from inevitable changes or inner work.

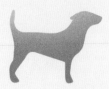

DOG

Known as man's best friend, the dog is a symbol of loyalty, faith, devotion, protection, trust, and companionship. Look for these qualities (or a lack thereof) in yourself or in those around you. Oftentimes, seeing a dog in a dream relates to matters of safeguarding or self-defense. Reflect on any areas of life that you feel emotionally protective over.

Dogs operate on instincts. Do you trust your instincts to guide you? Use your senses to "sniff out" a person's intentions before taking a leap of faith.

Pay attention to the color, shape, size, demeanor, breed, age, and actions of the dog to reveal underlying clues. For instance, dreaming of a puppy could imply that you're feeling protective over a new situation or relationship, while an older dog could represent a more established area of life or past attachment.

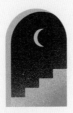

DOOR OR DOORWAY

A door serves as a passageway from one place to another.
Whether entering a new space or opportunity or exiting a
toxic situation, doors offer a powerful transition point to
change. While doors are usually thought of as portals of
expansion, they can also represent barriers, boundaries,
privacy, control, or protection. When encountering a door
in a dream, consider what you're moving toward as well
as what you're leaving behind.

Is the door open, closed, or
locked? The state of the door
may reveal your receptivity
or apprehension to changes
in life. An open door may
signify acceptance of these
changes, while a closed door
could indicate a blockage or
resistance.

A door can lead to anywhere,
which speaks to opportunities, potential, and choices.
Review your current options
wisely before making a final
decision. Remember, you
don't always have to open a
door. Sometimes it's better
to walk away.

DRIVING AN OUT-OF-CONTROL VEHICLE

A dream about driving an out-of-control car or other vehicle could mean that you do not feel in control of your own life. It implies that something is getting out of hand—whether a relationship, job, or addiction.

———

As the person behind the wheel, you are the one who is causing yourself to run off the tracks. Examine any subconscious influences that are "steering" your life in the wrong direction, including self-sabotaging behavior. Assess the ways you can regain control.

———

Are you driving too fast or recklessly? This could be a sign that you are acting carelessly and need to slow down. Rushing may indicate that you are pushing yourself to dangerous limits or placing yourself in risky situations.

FALLING

Falling dreams may speak to a sense of helplessness, anxiety, or loss of control in your waking life. The feeling of suddenly being thrown off balance may indicate that instabilities, insecurities, or a fear of failure are causing you to lose your footing in some respect.

———

Do you feel capable of supporting yourself? Can you stand on your own two feet? Dreaming of falling may be a sign that you feel inadequate or inferior in some capacity. Determine where these feelings are stemming from and ways you can strengthen your sense of self.

———

Because falling often happens by accident or surprise, this could signify that you are moving too fast or being careless with your plans. Are you missing any details? Take a moment to slow down and get your bearings. Performing your due diligence can help you avoid potential pitfalls.

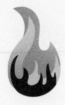

FIRE

Fire has the power to create as well as destroy. It can spark ideas into existence or reduce entire structures to ash. Seeing fire in a dream may speak to positive qualities such as passion, inspiration, and power, but it can also represent impulsivity, anger, or destruction. Consider the ways that you tend to your inner flame. How can you constructively channel your energy and emotions?

——

Observe the nature of the fire and the sensations it evokes. Is it a strong burning flame, dwindling embers, or a rapidly growing wildfire? Is it a source of warmth or danger? How the fire appears in your dream may mirror your drive, assertiveness, or feelings.

Pay attention to any items that are being burned. They may symbolize a situation or part of you that needs to be transformed. Being burned by fire could represent a burning desire within yourself or repressed feelings that need to be released. Fire can be used to purify, so take this opportunity to let go of anything that is no longer serving you.

FLYING

Dreams about flying are generally seen in a positive light. The ability to soar through the sky represents freedom and new perspectives and may serve as a reminder that anything is possible. Flying can have many functions, so think of the reasons why you might take flight. Are you flying to rise above obstacles, elevate your spiritual connection, or escape from certain stressors?

Flying may relate to your sense of control over a situation or level of confidence. Do you feel on top of your current affairs? Pay attention to the direction, speed, and altitude of your flight for insight. Flying at a slower speed or lower height could indicate that a project is still making its way off the ground, while flying backward could mean that you're feeling nostalgic about the past.

When you're flying, the sky's the limit! An unobstructed flight can symbolize hope and new possibilities. If you've been thinking about taking a leap of faith or considering a change of pace, now may be the time to spread your wings.

FOOD OR DRINK

Eating or drinking in a dream may represent a "hunger" or "thirst" in your waking life that needs to be fulfilled. Both food and drink provide nourishment to the body and are essential for life, so such dreams may be encouraging you to focus on your basic needs. Think about what fuels you on a mental, emotional, physical, and spiritual level. Have you been giving yourself the ingredients to not just survive, but thrive?

———

The type of food or drink you encounter, the way it tastes, and how it is consumed are highly relevant. Is it nutritious and healthy or full of empty calories? Did it make you feel satiated or sick? All of these are clues that may speak to the habits or behaviors you're currently developing or integrating into your life. Reflect on how these things contribute to your overall well-being.

———

Food or drink can symbolize thoughts, beliefs, or ideas that you are trying to "digest." Some information and truths can be hard to process. If something isn't sitting well, you may want to review whether it's providing the right kind of sustenance.

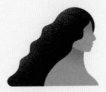

HAIR

Hair possesses powerful symbolism and may relate to themes of strength, self-image, health, and vitality. Some cultures consider hair to be an extension of one's spirit, soul, or life force. Since hair is often connected to personality and identity, think about what its outer attributes— such as its length, color, texture, and quality—may be saying about how you internally perceive yourself.

Psychoanalyst Sigmund Freud believed that losing hair was tied to anxiety over the aging process, while others thought this signified a loss of power or control. Whatever the case, think about any internalized anxiety or restrictive feelings you're experiencing in waking life that may be affecting your self-esteem or freedom.

Long, flowing hair is typically seen as a positive sign, indicating that you feel strong, attractive, and healthy. If your hair changes color in your dream, look to the meaning of that color for additional insight. For instance, red symbolizes passion, blue represents calming, and white speaks to cleansing or wisdom.

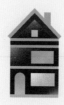

HOUSES OR BUILDINGS

Houses and buildings are often a reflection of your inner or outer world and may represent everything from your physical health to your emotional foundation. Noticing the condition, size, and location of the structure will tell you a lot about how you perceive yourself and your current state of affairs.

———

Does the house or building appear run-down or brand new? A derelict house could indicate that you've been neglecting to care for some aspect of life, while a new one may represent major changes that are taking place. A house that is under construction could mean that your plans are moving forward but that there is still more work to do.

———

Observe the size of the house, its style, and how it makes you feel. A cramped or outdated home may relate to feeling stifled or stuck in the past, while a spacious or modern home could symbolize a fresh mindset or room for growth. Think about how you've "constructed" your life up until now and what areas may be in need of a tune-up or redesign.

LATE

Dreams about being late for something usually speak to an opportunity that you feel like you've missed out on or an underlying anxiety in your waking life.

———

Being late for work or school may represent a lack of preparedness or self-discipline. This could be a sign that you've been acting irresponsibly and are internalizing some guilt. Take a moment to review your priorities and create a plan to get back on track.

Evaluate your current expectations. Are you being too critical of yourself? This type of dream can manifest from a pressure to achieve a desired result and may reflect your inner dissatisfaction with something. Although you may feel like you're "falling behind," this sentiment is often self-imposed. Take a moment to shift your perspective and acknowledge your progress thus far.

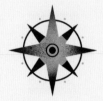

LOST

A dream of being lost suggests that you are feeling uncertain about your current direction in life or disconnected from a part of yourself. It may also point to an unfamiliar situation that you are attempting to navigate, which may be causing confusion, doubt, or anxiety.

———

Have you strayed from your authentic self recently? This type of dream may be a sign that you haven't been acting in alignment with your true nature or instincts. Consider what may be leading you astray, and whether you've become too dependent on others for guidance.

———

What is your destination in the dream? Recognizing where you are trying to go can show you where in your life you may be feeling lost. Getting lost on your way to work could point to an insecurity about your career path, while getting lost on your way home may indicate a weakened sense of self or lack of inner purpose.

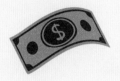

MONEY

While dreams about money may pertain to your finances, their meaning often extends beyond material possessions. At its core, money represents value and resources. Your sense of self-worth and self-esteem may be highlighted in these dreams, as well as what you spend your time, energy, and love on. Have you been investing your resources wisely? Take a moment to reevaluate your assets and priorities.

———

Notice the condition of the money, its location, quantity, and how you found it. New or crisp bills may symbolize success in your current endeavors, while old or crumpled ones could be a sign to look for new opportunities. Finding money in a hidden safe could represent untapped abilities within you that are ready to be unlocked.

———

Losing money in a dream may speak to a loss or setback in your waking life. This could be a close connection with a loved one, a business opportunity, or a situation that made you feel powerless. In moments like these, it's important to remember your intrinsic worth.

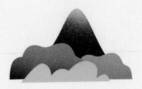

MOUNTAINS

In general, mountains are associated with overcoming obstacles, but they can also symbolize a union with nature, higher consciousness, or an enlightened point of view. Climbing a mountain in a dream may reveal that you're working toward a goal that requires committed effort and determination.

———

If you had difficulty ascending the mountain, was it because of the terrain, your technique, or your own fears? Consider the root of the issue, then reexamine your approach to the task at hand. Release any stubborn tendencies. Sometimes changing direction or learning a new skill is necessary to reach your destination.

———

Observe the size and shape of the mountain for clues to an obstacle's complexity. A small or gently sloping mountain could mean that a problem is easily manageable, while a steep or treacherous one could imply that extra caution and consideration are needed.

PARALYSIS

Dreams of being paralyzed typically point to some aspect of your life where you feel "pinned down" or restricted. The inability to move could be caused by underlying fears or anxieties, trappings of the past, limiting beliefs, or a loss of control. If you're feeling stuck in a situation, reflect on what is preventing you from moving forward. Is it possible that you're trapped in a prison of your own design?

Is your whole body paralyzed, or only certain parts? Look to the function of these parts to understand where blockages may be occurring. A paralyzed tongue may represent a communication issue or difficulty expressing your truth, while a paralyzed spine could speak to a lack of flexibility or support.

Pay attention to the setting of your dream for greater context. For instance, being paralyzed at work could relate to feeling stagnant in your career, while being paralyzed in front of a large crowd could relate to social or performance-based anxiety.

PHONE

Dreaming about a phone can speak to themes of communication, self-expression, connection, and information. Consider what you've been "calling" into your life recently and whether you've been listening to your inner voice.

———

Encountering a ringing phone may be highlighting an objective that needs your attention or an issue you've been ignoring. It could also be a sign that a message or spirit is trying to get through to you. Meditate to open up channels of communication.

———

A broken or malfunctioning phone may represent a communication issue. Has something gotten lost in translation? Do you feel a need to clear the air? This could also mean that you feel disconnected from someone close to you. Be mindful of the words you choose and how you "get through" to others.

PREGNANCY

Being pregnant in a dream symbolizes an aspect of yourself that is currently developing. This could be a new project, an idea, or a goal that you are birthing into existence. Dreams of pregnancy may be accompanied by feelings of excitement or anxiety, depending on how you feel about your growth. Are you ready for this new stage of expansion or are looming responsibilities weighing heavy on your mind?

———

Pregnancy may reflect the creative process. What "new life" are you bringing into being? Think about any intentions you've recently planted and how you've nourished their growth. Are you committed to seeing them flourish?

———

Difficulty with a pregnancy or birth may be a metaphor for obstacles that are blocking your creative expression. They could also signify that your ideas may need more time to germinate before they come to fruition.

ROBBERY OR HOME INVASION

Dreaming of a robbery or home invasion is often a metaphor for your private life. There may be something threatening your sense of security or privacy or encroaching upon your personal life. While this could be another person or party, don't discount feelings, habits, or obligations that have "taken over" in some regard, such as negative self-talk or spending too much time at work.

_____

Who or what is doing the invading in your dream? Understanding your relationship to the perpetrator(s) can inform you of subconscious fears and hidden issues. For instance, a stranger could represent fear of the unknown while a coworker or boss could indicate anxiety surrounding your career.

_____

This type of dream could be a sign that some boundary in your life is being violated. Has anyone crossed a line recently? Consider whether others have imposed their thoughts, beliefs, or feelings on you and how you can better protect your energy.

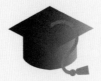

SCHOOL

A dream of a school or classroom suggests that there is a life lesson that you need to learn. If could also imply that you are learning something important about yourself. Raise your awareness of any negative behaviors, patterns, or habits that are keeping you stuck in past cycles so that you can evolve beyond them.

———

Is a situation in your current life "testing" you? Consider what the best way to approach it may be. Addressing the issue intentionally will help you feel more prepared to handle it.

———

This type of dream may symbolize a concern or an anxiety that is weighing heavily on your mind. The level of difficulty of the school may mirror how serious the issue is. For instance, an elementary school may reflect a general concern, while a college may represent something much more important or urgent.

SEX

Dreams about sex can be interpreted many ways. The person(s) and feelings involved are important pieces to review. If you engaged in sex with another person, consider what they may symbolize rather than how you feel about them personally. For instance, sex with a boss may point to acknowledging your own ambition or embracing your inner authority.

———

Sex is symbolic of union and may signify profound self-love or self-acceptance. You may be embracing, merging, or integrating different aspects of yourself, or knowledge outside of yourself, into your being. Take a moment to recognize your multifaceted nature and consider how to bring these sides of yourself into harmony.

———

Was the sex passionate or slow? Did it feel healing or liberating? The nature of the sex may represent energies that you wish to call into your life or your current relationship to pleasure. In a more straightforward sense, dreams about sex may simply be a manifestation of your primal desires.

SNAKE

Historically, snakes have been associated with regeneration, transformation, rebirth, fertility, and healing. This is largely due to their shedding process. Snakes shed their skin to allow for further growth and to remove parasites attached to their old skin. They may also shed their skin before reproduction or after giving birth. That said, seeing a snake in a dream may be highlighting themes related to personal growth and spiritual renewal in your life.

———

Consider the old habits, limiting beliefs, and outdated ways of thinking that are keeping you small. What do you need to "shed" or release before you can evolve? Keep in mind, purging old traumas and wounds can come with growing pains.

———

Examine any shifts in your life, whether positive or negative, especially those related to health and healing. Snakes can be poisonous, but their venom is also used to create medicine. Are you transforming your pain into a source of power and healing?

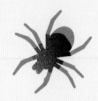

SPIDER

Spiders are often portrayed in a sinister light, but seeing one in your dreams isn't necessarily something to fear. Although spiders can represent darkness, looming anxieties, control issues, and manipulation, they're also symbols of creativity, ingenuity, productivity, and divine feminine power. So, are you stuck in a web of lies or weaving the web of your dreams? Search your feelings to find out.

———

Spiders are stealthy hunters, so be mindful of any manipulation or self-deception that may be taking place. Subconscious fears are like invisible strings. Be sure to cut loose from anything, or anyone, that makes you feel trapped.

———

Spiders are associated with the number eight due to the shape of their body and their eight legs. In numerology, this number is a symbol of creation and infinite possibilities. What thoughts, projects, or ideas are you weaving into existence? Are you designing your life in a way that will attract what you want?

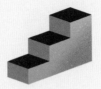

STAIRS, ELEVATOR, OR ESCALATOR

Stairs, elevators, and escalators are associated with themes of mobility and growth. Seeing any of them in a dream could mean that you're trying to reach a different level of consciousness or standing within your personal or professional life. Pay attention to the direction of movement within your dream for greater insight.

Upward movement is often linked to positive advancement (whether financially, spiritually, or socially), improvement in mood, new ideas and goals, or heightened awareness. Difficulty ascending could symbolize challenges along your path that you must overcome.

Conversely, downward movement could represent a loss of some sort, such as losing a valuable contract or falling out of touch with certain friends or groups. However, a downward journey isn't always negative. A descent can be symbolic of many things, like stepping down from a position that no longer resonates with you, grounding your energy, tending to your foundational needs, or delving more deeply into your subconscious.

TEETH

Teeth are a symbol of power. Used to bite, tear, and chew, they relate to your personal strength, confidence, and abilities. While they are not as unique as a fingerprint, they can be used to identify a person and, therefore, may be tied to themes surrounding ego or personal appearance.

––––

Losing teeth in a dream may point to a loss of power. Perhaps you are undergoing a period of change or personal loss that is throwing your life out of balance. Notice where any feelings of powerless-ness are stemming from and determine how you can reclaim your sovereignty. If you're worried about how others perceive you, practic-ing self-care may help.

––––

Teeth falling out may reflect a communication or health issue. If you've been gossiping or have spoken out of turn, this could be a sign to use your words more carefully. Losing teeth may also indicate that you've been neglecting your self-care routine.

TEST

Dreams about taking a test may be connected to anxiety. There may be a situation in your current life that you feel unprepared to handle, or you may be lacking confidence in your own abilities. Oftentimes, this type of dream indicates that an aspect of yourself has come under scrutiny. What are you judging and is the self-criticism warranted?

——

Dreams about test taking can highlight performance anxiety. Do you feel like you're measuring up? High expectations at work or home may be causing undue stress. Take a few minutes to review your goals and determine whether they're realistic and whether you're pursuing them at a sustainable pace.

——

Passing an exam symbolizes advancement, while failing one may be perceived as a setback. In this sense, dreams about taking an exam could manifest when you are attempting to progress to the next stage of your life. Being unprepared for the test or having difficulty answering questions may point to uncertainty surrounding these transitions. Look for obstacles, particularly mental ones, that may be obscuring your path forward.

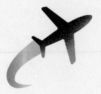

TRAVELING

Dreams of traveling are characterized by movement. The journey that you take, whether by car, plane, bus, bike, train, or boat, symbolizes the direction of your life path and the current progress you are making. Observe the type of vehicle you are traveling in and the landscape of the terrain for deeper insight.

———

Traveling through air may speak to an intellectual journey, while voyaging at sea could indicate an emotional journey. Traveling by land may relate to a physical journey or material changes, such as a new career or health routine.

———

Notice the appearance of your vehicle and how it performs, as these qualities may reflect your mental state. A fast-moving vehicle could signify that you are making significant progress, while a slow, old, or broken vehicle may imply that there is something impeding your growth. The latter could also point to feeling hesitant or uncertain about the direction you are heading in.

WATER

Water is symbolic of purity, fertility, fluidity, change, cleansing, healing, renewal, and life. It is considered the element of the unconscious and intuition. Water in dreams often represents your emotions in waking life. As a basic human need, water may speak to what you need emotionally in order to feel nourished.

———

From a serene lake to a tumultuous sea, water can be both soothing and terrifying. Pay attention to the form and location of water in your dreams (puddle, swimming pool, ocean, river, etc.), as each reveals different meanings.

———

Examine the water's movement and how it flows for clues to your subconscious emotional state. For instance, being lost on a stormy sea could be interpreted as having mixed or conflicting feelings that are hard to navigate, while a shower may represent a desire for self-renewal or washing away the past.

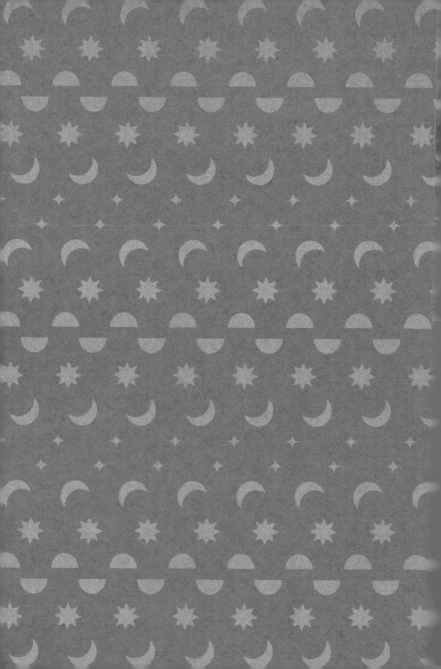